The Wizard of Oz Guide to Correctional Nursing

The Wizard of Oz Guide to Correctional Nursing is a creative and fun approach to delivering the basics about correctional health care. Lorry skillfully takes us on a parallel journey through Oz and the unique specialty of correctional nursing. As the reader navigates through the book, practical and relevant advice is offered. Novice and experienced correctional nurses will be reminded to stay focused, like Dorothy, on the ultimate goal of reaching Kansas. Kansas, for correctional nurses, is attained by providing great patient care through specialty knowledge, safety, and sound nursing practice. The comparison of the two worlds subtly delivers the message that each nurse holds the power to positively impact care delivery and patient lives.

Jennifer Slencak, BSN, RN, CCHP-RN
Correct Care Solutions
Corporate Director of Nursing – Corrections
Nashville, TN

I have been working as an RN nurse manager at a county jail for 3 years. Having not received any real orientation into the field of correctional nursing, finding books like this have been a Godsend! I have frequent staff turnover and think that this shall become a required reading during orientation. Nothing truly prepares you for the experiences you will have in this field of nursing but it certainly helps to have some information to get you through the fundamentals that we all seem to experience in our day to day work. Thank you so much for writing such an informative guide and what a wonderful way of relating it to my favorite movie of all times! It is so very relatable.

Becky Whitfill, RN
Macon County Jail
Decatur, IL

I have been a correctional nurse for 15 years and when I first stepped into the life of correctional nurse I wished I had a resource book such as this one that I could have referred to. Correctional nursing is such a specialty in itself that requires a certain learning curve that is obtained through years of experience. I would suggest that every nurse going into this field read "The Wizard of Oz Guide to Correctional Nursing" and keep one on their unit for reference.

Heather Robere RN
Central Nova Scotia Correctional Center
Dartmouth Nova Scotia Canada

I am constantly asked, "How is it working as a nurse in a prison?" This book is a must read for any nurse who is considering entering the correctional specialty or anyone with a curiosity as to what we have to deal with. It would also assist the community health care providers such as paramedics, emergency staff, and those working in community clinics and hospitals to understand what our capabilities and limitations are in a correctional setting. More importantly, it is a great reference and review for nurses who are already in this field. *Melani de la Vega, RN*
Correctional Case Manager
California State Prison Solano
Vacaville, CA

This book would be an excellent resource in nursing school (where so little is ever taught about corrections anyway and usually by tutors who have no idea of the reality of the day to day life of the correctional nurse). Even coming from another country and another Correctional and Justice system this book draws strong parallels and is a must read for the new correctional nurse just starting out. There are also suggestions and concepts that can form mind mapped connections for later use! A straight forward and easy read. Thank you for this publication, Lorry!

Helen Hendren
BN, NZRN
Department of Corrections (NZ)

The Wizard of Oz Guide to Correctional Nursing: This Isn't Kanas Anymore, Toto! reflects the journey to becoming a Correctional Nurse. Dr. Lorry Schoenly is certainly the wizard helping us thru Oz. This is exactly the resource that has been missing from the world of correctional nursing. I found it to be clearly written which will enable the new, as well as the seasoned, correctional nurse the ability to navigate the medical, mental health, moral, and legal issues that arise in a correctional institution. This book addresses the medical and mental health conditions particular to Correctional Nursing (such as Taser, pepper spray, and suicides), then gives the health care management and actions to be taken. This book will be a tool that I will use to retaining new hires so they will not be lost on the yellow brick road to Oz!!!

Kathleen Cannon, RN DON
Cumberland County Department of Corrections
Bridgeton, NJ

This book is the recipe for success in corrections nursing. Everything I wish I'd known in the first year is here. A wonderful reference for those training new medical staff.

K. Paige Ridenour, LPN, C/O
Washington County Jail
Marietta, OH

From protecting your body, your mind, your reputation, and your license to prison ink and Hepatitis B & C, Lorry covers it all here in The Wizard of Oz Guide to Correctional Nursing. A must read for all nurses new to corrections and seasoned nurses, as well. When you discover that someone has just put your passion for correctional nursing into print, you will be unable to put it down.

Melissa Donahue RN
Illinois Dept. Of Corrections, Danville

Very good information. I wish I had a book like this when I began my nursing career in corrections. Will be very helpful to new nurses entering the correctional setting.

D. Birchmore, LPN
Tyger River Correctional Institution
Enoree, SC

What an interesting and informative read!! I'm relatively new to the wild world of corrections nursing and have learned a few things the hard way! Like Dorothy in Oz, I quickly learned that things are not always what they seem. Correctional health staff need to remember that they are on the HEALTH side of the coin, not the PUNISHMENT side!

Katharine Marker, RN
Miami County Sheriff's Office
Clinic Coordinator

I love your new book! Nurses new to corrections will have a better understanding of the importance of correctional nursing and that our role in nursing is just as important as that of our colleagues in hospitals and clinics. Those of us who have several years of experience will be able to relate to some of the situations described and can do a mental review of what to do differently or better. We all learn little tricks like keeping ammonia inside chem-strip containers and bandage scissors in your pen pocket for suicide cut-downs. We do make a difference and I have actually been thanked outside the wall by some of my former patients for my part in "cleaning up their acts." I intend to get a few copies of the book to pass around!

Chris Ledding, LPN, CCHP
Advanced Correctional Healthcare
Owensboro, KY

Phenomenal book!! Learned a lot for being a seasoned correctional nurse. I can see this book being used as a training requirement for new and seasoned nurses. Looking forward to reading more from you!

Pete Briggs – LPN
Nurse Trainer and Infectious Disease instructor
Maine Correctional Center, Windham, Maine

The Wizard of Oz Guide to Correctional Nursing, This Isn't Kansas Anymore, Toto! is a great resource for the new nurse who is trying to navigate the specialty world of corrections nursing. It provides a good balance of general information, like what to anticipate working in a setting where healthcare is secondary to security, as well which medical and mental disorders are more prevalent and how to properly assess and manage care for this population. As a current corrections nurse, I found it equally informative and a great refresher especially regarding the legal implications in working in a corrections setting. It's taken me almost two years to gain the knowledge the author, Lorry Schoenly, details so clearly for a new nurse.

Michelle B. Valencia-Stark, RN
Bernalillo County Metropolitan Detention Center
Albuquerque, NM

I thoroughly enjoyed this book! As an experienced correctional nurse I believe this book brings vital information to any correctional nurse, both experienced and inexperienced. This book gives invaluable insight to the new correctional nurse in a relatable way that sparks interest and makes the information easy to both understand and apply to real world scenarios. The pictures add an extra layer to the information that provides a visual explanation of things that might be difficult to imagine. Overall, this is an excellent book!

Nicole Lane, RN, ADON
Arizona State Prison Complex
Tucson, AZ

This is a wonderful book full of valuable information for anyone in the correctional nursing field. Correctional nursing takes a special type of person. I suggest anyone working in this field or potentially interested to check out this book.

Andrea Adams LPN
NEOCC, Ohio

The Wizard of Oz Guide to Correctional Nursing: This Isn't Kansas Anymore, Toto! is a concise tutorial that quells the baptism by fire nurses transitioning into corrections experience. A quick and insightful read that will assist newer nurses to navigate the unique challenges faced working in the correctional setting, while offering perspective and helping to guard against desensitization for more seasoned professionals. This book is a must read for nurses entering the correctional work force and a necessary item for nurse managers hoping to decrease turnover and create nurses equipped to handle anything they may encounter inside the walls.

Katie Schmidt, BA, BSN, RN, CCN
Kansas Juvenile Correctional Complex
Topeka, Kansas

Once again, you have addressed a need in correctional nursing. I wish I had this resource when I first walked through those metal gates 12 years ago! The basic understanding of the working environment, culture, security requirements and diverse health care needs of our patients was not something that any of us thinks about when thinking of our career goals. Having said that, I learned even more than my years in corrections has taught me, some of the terminology is new to me and the legal aspects also gave some insight and new knowledge. Thank you for continuing to lead us in the "building of the cathedral", I will continue to work towards that goal along with you and all of my correctional nursing colleagues.

Denise R Rahaman, MBA, BSN, CCHP-RN
Director of Operations CFG Health Systems.
Multiple County Jails in NJ

The Wizard of Oz Guide to Correctional Nursing will benefit new and experienced registered nursing by gaining the much needed information to continue supplying our patient base with quality care. As a brand new nurse starting out in correctional healthcare, the needs of inmates with mental health and physical issues; that are many times a direct cause of substance abuse, has been very challenging. Providing healthcare to individuals that have spent the vast majority of their lives indulging in substances that have had a detrimental effect on their overall body systems has forced me as a brand new registered nurse to make instant life-saving decisions based upon the unknown. With the continual turnover of inmate populations it is imperative as a new registered nurse to continue with all forms of education that are focusing on this patient type.

Shelly R Davis, RN, BSN, PHN
California Forensic Medical Group
Butte County Jail
Oroville, CA

The Wizard of Oz Guide to Correctional Nursing

This Isn't Kansas Anymore, Toto!

Other books by Lorry Schoenly

Correctional Health Care Patient Safety Handbook

The Correctional Nurse Manifesto

Essentials of Correctional Nursing

The Wizard of Oz Guide to Correctional Nursing

This Isn't Kansas Anymore, Toto!

Lorry Schoenly
PhD, RN, CCHP-RN
Correctional Health Care Risk Consultant
Visiting Professor
Chamberlain College of Nursing
Graduate Nursing Program
Downers Grove, IL

Enchanted Mountain Press

The Wizard of Oz Guide to Correctional Nursing
This isn't Kansas Anymore, Toto!

Copyright © 2015 Lorry Schoenly

CorrectionalNurse.Net

All rights reserved.

No part of this publication may be reproduced, stored in a retrieval system, or transmitted in any form or by any means, electronic, mechanical, photocopying, recording, or otherwise without the prior permission of the copyright holder. Please contact lorry@correctionalnurse.net for permission or special discounts on bulk quantities.

Published in the United States by Enchanted Mountain Press

ISBN: 978-0-9912942-7-5

Every effort has been made to use sources believed to be reliable to provide this information. The author and publisher shall not be liable for any special, consequential, or exemplary damages resulting, in whole or in part, from the readers' use of, or reliance on, the information contained in this book.

Contents

Introduction – Caught in a Tornado	i
SECTION I This isn't Kansas Anymore, Toto!	**1**
Chapter 1: A Different Work Environment	3
Chapter 2: A Different Patient Population	7
Chapter 3: A Different Language	13
Chapter 4: Different Types of Colleagues	17
Chapter 5: Same Dorothy, Though	21
SECTION II If I Only Had a Brain – Correctional Nurse Knowledge	**25**
Chapter 6: Health Care Processes	27
Chapter 7: High Risk Issues	43
Chapter 8: Unusual Medical Conditions	53
Chapter 9: Frequent Mental Health Issues	65
Chapter 10: The Women and Children	85
Chapter 11: Correctional Nurse Legal Concerns	95
SECTION III More than an Empty Tin Chest – Correctional Nurse Caring	**109**
Chapter 12: Caring in the Correctional Environment	111
Chapter 13: Working with Inmates as Patients	117
Chapter 14: Guarding Your Heart and Person	123
SECTION IV The Nerve – Courage to be a Correctional Nurse	**133**
Chapter 15: Moral Courage in the Correctional Context	135
SECTION V Destination – Emerald City and the Wizard	**145**
Chapter 16: Who is in Charge Here?	147
Conclusion – You Have Always Had the Power!	**153**
About the Author	157
References	159

Introduction – Caught in a Tornado

Nursing in a jail, prison, or juvenile detention facility is very different from nursing in a traditional setting. Indeed, many nurses feel just like Dorothy Gale from the Wizard of Oz tale walking out into the Land of Oz when her prairie home landed on the Wicked Witch of the East following a tornado ride from Kansas. Seeing officers, handcuffs, sally ports, and metal detectors can easily bring to mind Dorothy's admonition to her little dog that "This isn't Kansas anymore, Toto!" It is easy, then, to get confused as to who you are as a nurse and what you are doing here behind bars. But it doesn't have to be this way. With the information in this guide, you can power down that Yellow Brick Road and feel at home in the Land of Oz before you know it.

This book started as a keynote address to correctional nurse managers from Correct Care Solutions in the fall of 2014. As I pondered the meaning of working in our specialty and considered the many things I wanted to say to inspire and motivate these wonderful nurse managers, I happened upon a notice of the Wizard of Oz movie's 75th anniversary that year. In a flash, I realized that Dorothy in the Land of Oz was a perfect framework to unpack the many facets of working in our specialty. Whether new to corrections or a seasoned jail or prison nurse, the information ahead can help you to provide competent and compassionate professional nursing in the criminal justice system.

As a practical guide, this book is written informally, and even light-heartedly, to be of maximum applicability for the practicing front-line correctional staff nurse. I did not clutter the writing with citations but references used for this book are listed at the conclusion. Much of the material comes from blog posts I have written over the last five years on the CorrectionalNurse.Net blog. So, come along on a journey to the Land of Oz and down the Yellow Brick Road to find, like Dorothy, that there is no place like home. In this case, you will be seeking to find your home in the specialty of correctional nursing!

SECTION I

This isn't Kansas Anymore, Toto!

When a tornado swept Dorothy's Kansas home into the air, she landed over the rainbow in the Land of Oz. Dorothy knew right away that the land she stepped into was not Kansas. You can be sure that a jail or prison is very different from other nursing experiences you have had. Stepping into the correctional world can be disorienting. The work environment, patient population, language spoken, and work colleagues in correctional nursing practice are unique. This section explores these differences.

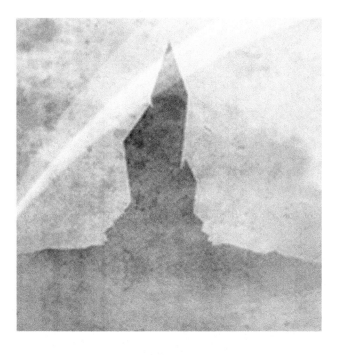

Chapter 1: A Different Work Environment

"She was hungry! Well, how would you like to have someone come along and pick something off of you?" – Apple Tree

"Oh dear! I keep forgetting I'm not in Kansas!" – Dorothy Gale

Dorothy had to keep reminding herself that she was not in Kansas. There were different rules of living and interacting in this new Land of Oz. As she walked along the Yellow Brick Road, she felt hungry and assumed she could pick apples from the trees along the side of the road as she would have done in the same situation in Kansas. Not so, as she soon found out! Apple trees in the Land of Oz talk and are possessive of their fruit. Correctional nurses need to know and understand their particular work environment. As you will see, it comes with different rules and goals as well.

A particular correctional health care work environment is based on the location within the criminal justice system. Here is an overview of the key concepts of the system. As you review the elements of this work environment, consider where your facility or intended facility of employment fits into the system.

Detained vs. Sentenced

Depending on the setting and geographic location, security staff use several terms for the correctional population. For example, in a jail setting, those who have not been sentenced for a crime may be referred to as "arrestees" or "detainees". While in some areas, those in a jail or prison setting who have been convicted may be called "offenders". A common general term for individuals in any area of the criminal justice system is "inmate". This is the best term for referring to the patient population in general. When referring to an inmate in a health care relationship, however, it is best to use the term "patient".

Those in the criminal justice system may be there as detainees awaiting arraignment and charges or they may be awaiting their court hearing or trial. In some places they are called "pre-sentence" or "pretrial" inmates. "Sentenced" inmates are those who have been convicted of a violation of law that requires incarceration.

Jails and Prisons

It is important to know the difference between a jail and a prison when considering the health care needs of the incarcerated patient population.

Jails

Jails are short-term detention facilities that house individuals booked in on probable cause for committing a crime. They may be awaiting a court case or bail. Jails can also house those convicted of a crime with sentences lasting less than 12 months. Rather than move them to the prison system, they serve out their sentence in the jail location. Jails are managed by county or city government. Individuals are booked in to the jail through an intake process that includes a health screening. The temporary and transient nature of the jail setting affects health care delivery. Inmates come in directly "off the street" so there can be great concern for alcohol and drug withdrawal. Stabilizing any health condition is a priority in this setting.

Prisons

Prisons house individuals who have been convicted of a crime and are serving out their sentence. Inmates transfer in to a prison system from the jail system through a reception process that evaluates and classifies the individual as to health need, functionality, and security level. This information is used to determine placement in the prison system. Prisons provide more predictable ambulatory care and have a more long-term relationship with the patient population. Although inmates can be moved within the systems for security reasons, they will generally be in a long-term relationship with their care providers.

State Prison System. Those convicted of a state crime serve out their sentence in the state prison system. The states prosecute most crimes against the person, such as murders and assaults, and many crimes against property, such as robberies and thefts. Indeed, states prosecute a far greater number of crimes than does the federal government. Small states such as Delaware and Rhode Island have combined jail/prison facilities.

Federal Prison System. Those convicted of a federal crime serve out their sentence within the federal prison system. The Federal Bureau of Prisons includes over 100 facilities throughout the country where those convicted of such federal crime as drug trafficking, organized crime, large-scale fraud, or financial crimes serve out their sentence.

Prison or jail, sentenced or pretrial, no matter the status of your patients, it is best to avoid knowing about their criminal activities, other than security level. As health care professionals our ethical codes require us to establish a trusting patient relationship to deliver care. Knowing too much personal information can make it difficult to see the patient behind the criminal.

Health Care Delivery Models

There are several ways health care can be delivered in the criminal justice system. The two most common ways are self-operated and independent health care services. A small number of states, such as Connecticut and New Jersey, have inmate health care managed and delivered through their state university medical systems.

Governmental Agencies (Self-Operated)

Most correctional nurses work for the same employer as their custody peers. Currently, about fifty-eight (58) percent of correctional health care facilities are in this category. The industry calls this "self-operated" or "self-op". Health care managers in this management structure are a part of the organizational hierarchy and reporting framework. This can be a great advantage for making changes or obtaining resources as the health care manager is on parity with other services, therefore fostering support for inmate medical needs. There are disadvantages to this arrangement as well. Although the well-being of the inmate population is a common goal for both custody and nursing staff, professional frameworks and guiding principles can differ. Nurses in these organizations must be vigilant to maintain professional nursing judgment in all matters of care delivery.

Independent Health Care Service Companies

The next most frequent health care management structure is an independent health care company. Thirty (30) percent of correctional health care is provided through a contracted arrangement between the government entity and a health care company. Nurses are most often employees of the health care service company and report to managers within the company. In this situation, correctional nurses need to understand the contractual relationship with the corrections administration to know what may be required of them. For example, services may include providing health care to security staff and emergency treatment to visitors. Also important is an understanding of the communication and reporting structures among all the players. In this situation, nurses are guests in the facility and must strive to develop collaborative working relationships with custody staff.

State University Medical Systems

Several state prison systems provide health care to inmates through the state university system. Twelve (12) percent of correctional health care is delivered in this manner. For example, in Connecticut inmates receive care through the University of Connecticut medical system and in New Jersey health care services are provided through the state's medical education system. Nurses working in these systems have the advantage of access to academic resources while nursing, medical, and dentistry students have an opportunity to experience the correctional environment. The corollary in jails is that the county health department may provide the health care at the jail. In this situation, nurses have the advantage of access to the resources of the county health department. Although health care staff are not employees of the same entity as corrections staff, a common relationship exists among the government bodies.

Types of Health Care Provided

An efficient security system will maximize health care within the security perimeter in order to reduce the manpower needs and escape risk of transporting inmates to outside resources. Depending on the size and type facility, the following types of health care are delivered in a correctional medical unit.

- *Ambulatory Care* – Urgent care for acute conditions and ongoing chronic disease management similar to an office setting. Ambulatory dental services are also provided.

- *Emergency Care* – Evaluation of trauma and emergency symptoms, along with treatment of minor trauma.

- *Mental Health Services* – Treatment of major mental health illness, including psychiatric care and group therapy, is provided in larger facilities. Some systems are moving to telehealth to be able to provide increased access to mental health providers.

- *Sub-acute Care* – Management of short duration therapies such as IV antibiotics and wound management. In traditional health care, some of these conditions might be managed through homecare but require the use of equipment, such as IV needles, that are unsafe in the general inmate population.

- *Long-Term and End-of-Life Care* – Inmates incarcerated late in life or serving out long sentences need management of declining functionality or end-of-life care for terminal conditions. Some prison systems group these patients together to provide specialized services in a single facility.

Dorothy developed an understanding of the Land of Oz while on her journey to the Emerald City. Having an understanding of the criminal justice system will help you to better navigate the system as you deliver health care.

Chapter 2: A Different Patient Population

"Now I... I know we're not in Kansas!" – Dorothy Gale to Toto

The inhabitants of Munchkin Land were not like Dorothy's family and friends back home. Oh, sure, there were many similarities, but so many differences. Apple trees talk and monkeys fly in the Land of Oz. In many ways the patient population is very different in a correctional setting than back home at the hospital. The demographics of incarceration mean that correctional nurses are providing health care to vulnerable, marginalized patients with less health knowledge and less prior health care contact than those in traditional settings. Like Dorothy, correctional nurses must come to understand the characteristics of the citizens of this new land.

Characteristics of the Incarcerated Patient Population

Age

Although generally young and male, the inmate population is aging along with the general US population. Inmates, however, due in part to poor prior health care, stressful lifestyle, and poor self-care practices, seem to age faster biologically than chronologically. Many correctional systems consider any inmate over 50 to be elderly. These older inmates required increasing medical and mental health services.

Those under 18 years of age are most often designated as youth or juvenile in the correctional setting. The majority of juveniles are segregated from the adult incarcerated population in separate detention facilities. However, a growing number of youth are convicted under adult sentencing guidelines and end up in adult facilities. Understanding the elderly and youth populations in your facility will help in determining a plan of care.

Gender

The majority of the inmate population is male; however, the female inmate population is growing at a fast rate. Female inmates will be segregated from the male population in separate housing areas in a jail or in a separate prison within a state or federal system. Female inmates use medical and mental health services more frequently than male inmates. They have additional issues of pregnancy and reproductive cancers, and have high rates of past sexual and domestic abuse.

Race/Ethnicity

The inmate population is disproportionately black and Hispanic. Therefore, those conditions more prevalent in these ethnic groups are of increased concern in the correctional population. Black Americans have higher rates of diabetes and stroke than the general population. Black men have higher rates of HIV and lung, stomach, and colorectal cancers. Black women have higher rates of colon, pancreatic, and stomach cancers.

The Hispanic population has disproportionately higher rates of stroke, chronic liver disease, diabetes, and HIV disease than the general population. In addition, rates of stomach and cervical cancers are higher. This information can help to develop screening and treatment programs in correctional facilities.

Education

Generally, the inmate patient population has less education than the general patient population, with less than half graduating high school. They are also twice as likely to have learning disabilities and basic literacy is low. This has implications for patient teaching and for interpreting and understanding self-care direction provided in a patient encounter. When providing important health instruction, then, have the patient speak-back the information and explain what it means for what they need to do. This will confirm understanding or allow an opportunity to clarify a misunderstood point.

Physical Health

The inmate population presents a wide array of conditions similar to the general patient population. However, chronic and infectious disease is of particular concern when providing health care to this patient group.

Chronic Illness

Studies have found higher incidence of several chronic conditions in the inmate patient population. Special attention is needed to these diseases in the diagnosis and treatment plans of care providers. In addition, collaboration may be needed with correctional officers regarding chronic disease management. For example, officers may need to be aware of asthma and diabetes diagnosis if they are required to intervene in a respiratory or hypoglycemic episode. Patient education is a primary component of all chronic disease treatment plans as this patient population is less aware of disease management self-care.

Chapter 2: A Different Patient Population

Asthma. Asthma management in a secure setting is complicated by the potential inappropriate use of inhalers if allowed to be in the possession of the patient. Highly sensitive asthmatics may also react to environmental factors in the prison as many facilities are older with poor air circulation. Officers may need to be aware of an asthma diagnosis if chemical agents such as pepper spray are being contemplated.

Cardiovascular Disease. Higher levels of myocardial infarction and hypertension in this patient population will require attention. Medical management includes lipid control and antihypertensives with increased attention to patient education about the condition and lifestyle modifications that can be attained in the corrections environment. Patients may need focused attention with dietary selection, weight management, and obtaining adequate physical activity while confined. Practical help in developing a heart-healthy lifestyle is needed.

Diabetes. Diabetes management in the correctional setting is made difficult by limited, and often poor, food options in the facility menu and the commissary. Insulin administration must be managed around the security schedule as inmates are not provided syringes and needles for self-administration. Healthy lifestyle teaching is an important part of care delivery but attention to low literacy levels and learning disabilities is needed.

Infectious Diseases

This patient population is prone to higher rates of several infectious disease categories based on a background of substance abuse, risky sexual behaviors, lack of medical care and poor nutrition. Awareness of the higher likelihood of these conditions can lead to early detection and treatment. In addition, infection can spread quickly in a confined environment with inadequate attention to personal hygiene and transmission. Maintaining a high suspicion of infectious disease can lead to early containment and transmission disruption.

HIV and Hepatitis C. Blood-borne diseases like HIV and Hepatitis C are common in the inmate population. Intravenous drug use, risky sexual behaviors, and self-administered tattoos or piercings are widespread in this patient group.

Sexually Transmitted Infections. Similarly, instances of Chlamydia, Gonorrhea, and Syphilis are high in this group. The geographic location of the correctional facility may determine prevalence and standard treatment protocols.

Tuberculosis (TB). This infectious disease is of growing concern in the inmate population with an infection rate of at least three times that of the general public. Testing for TB should take place at intake and those with a suspicion of the condition should be isolated until the infection is ruled out.

Mental Health

Studies confirm that there are now more mentally-ill Americans incarcerated than in mental health facilities, making this a major correctional health care concern. More than half of all inmates reported having a recent mental health problem.

Mental Illness

Inmates have high rates of depression, mania, and psychotic disorders. In addition, a significant portion of the patient population has borderline personality disorders with characteristics of poor impulse control, self-injury, and substance abuse. These symptoms contributed to the crimes that result in incarceration and also contribute to potential aggression or boundary violation in the health care setting. For this reason, correctional health care workers need to be ever-vigilant when providing health care to inmates.

Traumatic Brain Injury/Post-Traumatic Stress Disorder

Due to a lifestyle of trauma, assault, and military duty, the inmate patient population has high rates of traumatic brain injury and post-traumatic stress disorder (PTSD). These conditions contribute to the already high rates of depression, anxiety, substance abuse, and poor anger management in this community. Female inmates, in particular, have frequent histories of childhood and domestic abuse that can lead to PTSD. Symptoms of this condition can affect patient care; and conditions of confinement such as loud, aggressive voice tones, enclosed areas, and perceived coercion can trigger unexpected reactions.

Drug/Alcohol/Tobacco Use

Substance abuse frequently co occurs with mental illness, making it particularly difficult to manage. A high suspicion of drug or alcohol involvement should be considered at all intake assessments and substance use should be part of the differential diagnosis in patient evaluations of altered mental states and acute emergencies, even after incarceration.

Those entering the correctional setting are frequently smokers. With more and more facilities moving to a smoke-free environment, this can lead to nicotine withdrawal symptoms. Nicotine withdrawal can exacerbate other withdrawal and confinement stresses such as abrupt elimination of access to drugs, alcohol, or pain treatment.

Suicidality

Attempted and completed suicide rates are much higher in the incarcerated population than the general public. Suicide potential should be considered for all

Chapter 2: A Different Patient Population

individuals entering a correctional facility. In addition, times of added stress such as when convicted, when family members withdraw (divorce notice), or when threated while in custody (such as rape, gang activity or personal violence) can lead to contemplation of self-harm. Be on the alert for indications of suicide potential in all correctional settings, but particularly jails.

Dorothy modified her thoughts and actions in the Land of Oz by realizing things were different. You can, too!

Chapter 3: A Different Language

"Are you a good witch, or a bad witch?" – Glinda, the Good Witch of the North

"I'm not a witch at all. I'm Dorothy Gale from Kansas." – Dorothy Gale

Dorothy thought she understood what was being said to her in Oz, but soon found out that things could have very different meanings. Jails and prisons have their own language and correctional nurses must understand what their patients and correctional colleagues are talking about to provide effective care. Here are some common words and phrases to get to know to help you to be an effective correctional nurse. Remember, though, that terms may vary depending on geography and work setting. For example, correctional nurses from all over the country were polled about what they call the slot in the cell door used to transfer items such as meals or to cuff the inmate before opening the door. Here are the various terms provided: Hatch, Trap, Flap, Trap door, Food Port, Food Slot, Chuck Hole, Pie Flap, Pie Hole, Bean Hole, Trap Port, Pan Hole, Feed-up Hatch, Hash Hole, Shute, Pass-Through, and Wicket.

So, although terms may be different depending on setting, here are some common terms used in correctional facilities by inmates and staff.

- *Ad-Seg* – Administration Segregation. Separate unit with increased security and decreased privileges. Separate from general population. In-custody penalty for fighting, causing disturbances, or being a danger to others.

- *AWO* – All the Way Out. Release from the facility.

- *Books* – An inmate's money account at the prison to buy certain items at the store, stamps, co-pays for medical.

- *Breakfast* – Legal speed, like coffee, Mt. Dew, yellow jackets.

- *Catch a Case or Get a Case* – Purposefully getting into trouble; for example, to prolong a death sentence or increase a stay in segregation that protects from other inmates. Can also mean receiving an internal penalty for wrong behavior – like being somewhere without a pass. Can affect parole hearing later.

- *Chaining Out/Chaining In* – Going to or coming from another location. The process that accompanies transportation across the security perimeter. In a medical situation, this requires a review of any new medical information. For instance, if they were transported to an acute care facility, whether associated with the prison or not.

- *Cheeking* – Hiding medication in the mouth for use later. Stockpiling for overdose or, more usually, for use as barter among inmates.

- *Chow* – Dining hall. Where the inmates eat.

- *C.O.* – Correctional Officer or Custody Officer. Never refer to these individuals as 'guards'. The correctional hierarchy follows the military or police format with officers, captains, sergeants, etc.

- *Code Brown* – Code for having to take a poop.

- *Code Red* – Lockdown. No movement in the facility.

- *Contraband* – Any item unacceptable for inmates to possess. Sharps, alcohol wipes, rubber bands, and cell phones are examples. Different listings for different populations.

- *Count or In Count* – Times of day when all traffic stops and an accurate count of inmates is taken. Everyone must be accounted for and in an approved location. CO's call in their count to a central location. Count has to match numbers of inmates assigned to their housing assignments. If an inmate is not where they are supposed to be according to their pass (i.e. medical or education or library) they are regarded as being "out of place", and can Get a Case (see above).

- *DOT* – Direct Observation Therapy – Inmate must come to a medication line and receive each dose of medication directly from the nurse. A custody officer checks that the medication is taken and swallowed (oral search).

- *Gen Pop* – General Population. The primary inmate community with the least limitations on movement and independence. Gen Pop inmates receive medications through a medication line process, usually can obtain KOP medications, and access health care services by submitting a request.

- *Keister* – Put contraband up one's rectum. May require an x-ray for validation.

- *Kite* – a sick call request written by an inmate to ask to see a health care provider. Also called 'a slip' as in 'drop a slip' to see the nurse.

- *KOP* – Keep on Person – Medication distributed monthly to inmates for self-administration. These are usually chronic medications. Pain medications, TB medications, and psychotropics are rarely approved for KOP distribution at a correctional facility.

Chapter 3: A Different Language

- *Lockdown* – Severe restriction of inmate movement for an urgent security need.
- *Man down* – Custody term for an inmate suffering from a medical issue that requires medical or nursing assessment and treatment in the yard, housing unit, or cell.
- *ODR* – Officer Dining Room – where the staff are served. In many facilities it is considered a prime place for inmates to work. Only inmates on good behavior and free of communicable diseases are awarded this post.
- *OPM* – On Person Med. See KOP above.
- *PC* – Protective Custody. Same as SHU, SNU. See below.
- *Racking Them Up* – All inmates sent back to cells or pods/bunks (if they live in a dorm) until further notice. Can happen prior to a Lockdown, if a Count was off and could not be explained by the records, for an out-of-control situation or security risk.
- *RTC* – Return to Custody. Inmate returns from an outside event such as a specialty appointment or the hospital.
- *Sally Port* – A double-door entryway into the facility or between areas within the facility among different levels of security. Only one door is allowed open at a time in a sally port so that there is never an open passage between the two sections. Doors are manually operated by officers.
- *SHU* – Special Housing Unit. Protective area for older inmates, openly gay inmates, sex offenders, people who drop from gangs – anyone who would be at risk of injury/retaliation if placed in general population.
- *SNU* – Special Needs Unit. See SHU above.
- *STG* – Security Threat Groups. Another term for gangs.
- *Taking a Sit-Down* – Having a bowel movement.
- *Ticket* – A report writing up an inmate for breaking the rules.
- *Yard down* – Medical or custody incident in the recreation yard requiring increased security. While the incident is managed, inmates must get down on the ground, either sitting or prone, depending on the institution.

In the Land of Oz, Dorothy discovered there are good witches and bad witches. This helped her navigate. Correctional nurses must understand the terms and abbreviations used by patients and colleagues to navigate their territory as well.

Chapter 4: Different Types of Colleagues

Whether a Scarecrow, a Tin Man, or a talking Lion, Dorothy's colleagues were also very different than she was used to. Her colleagues back home were just like her – humans of various sizes, shapes, and interests. On her journey to the Emerald City, she learned to be interested in avoiding fires for the scarecrow and keeping the oil can handy for the Tin Man. She and her colleagues all had the same goal – getting to the Wizard – but they each had a different reason and perspective. Correctional nurses find themselves among different types of colleagues in the land behind the security perimeter, too. Coming from a traditional health care setting managed by other health care professionals, the differences can quickly become apparent. Correctional officers don't think like health care professionals and correctional organizations are managed from a different perspective as well.

The primary service of every correctional facility is security. The primary concerns of correctional officers are for order, control, and discipline. These concerns support the goal of personal and public safety. Most correctional environments are organized in a para-military fashion and often use military rank designations. It is important, then, to respect these designations and order of command. Here is a quick listing of rank to help you determine the authority structure (highest to lowest): Chief, Major, Captain, Lieutenant, Sergeant, Corporal, Deputy/Officer. Of course, designations vary among systems and regions of the country so check out the officer titles in your specific facility and use them appropriately. Just remember that no one in a correctional facility is called a guard. This is a true sign of disrespect.

Communication and Collaboration

Working with custody in a secure environment such as a jail or prison requires additional communication and collaboration skill. Health care and security perspectives can be at odds in some situations. Security administration and officers focus on public safety (maintaining incarceration) and the personal safety of those in the facility (both staff and inmates). Health care staff, although also concerned about these issues, are ethically bound to seek the physical and mental well-being for individual patients and the patient population they serve. When these goals clash, negotiation is necessary to come to an agreement on the best course of action. Therefore, it is important to develop collegial, trusting relationships with the security officers and administrators in your facility.

Since custody officers are not health care providers, only patient medical information that is necessary for their role in managing the patient can be shared with them. Housing officers, for example, may need to know that a patient is diabetic and needs immediate attention if they request to be seen by medical. Also, a housing assignment may indicate a patient condition, such as when an inmate is assigned to the protective mental health unit.

One of the most difficult adjustments that correctional nurses must make is learning to work with security staff without sacrificing nursing perspective. Making the adjustment is often difficult, but it can be done.

Correctional personnel are like most people; they have preconceived notions about how nurses behave and think. Sometimes, correctional staff can be critical of nursing concepts like compassion and patient advocacy, but they still do not like it when nurses do not act as expected. Role modeling expected nurse behavior may invite some teasing, but generally the security staff will have greater respect for a nurse who is 'acting like one'.

Mutual respect will go a long way to facilitate collaboration with correctional staff. Officers and administrators have a hard job. Correctional nurses need to recognize this and refrain from being overly critical or judgmental about security perspectives about prisoners – while still maintaining a nursing perspective. Professional courtesy and consideration help when collaborating with security colleagues.

Avoid Going Native

Another challenge of working with correctional officers is that we can 'go native' and lose our professional nursing bearings; choosing, instead, to assimilate fully into the custody culture and identify with the security perspective over the health care perspective. Correctional officers often have different goals and worldviews than health care staff.

Researchers Hardesty, Champion, and Champion interviewed 26 registered and licensed practical nurses working in jails in three northern states. Patterns and themes emerged as the transcribed interviews were analyzed. One interesting finding was a proposed typology of jail nurse work styles. This typology chronicles the adjustment of a new nurse to the correctional culture and the effect of that adjustment on their ability to function successfully. The categories are based primarily on the balance that the nurse is able to gain practicing professionally while understanding the security perspective and organizational culture.

Check out this continuum of jail nurse work styles and see if you can find yourself, or some of your nurse colleagues, in the descriptions.

Chapter 4: Different Types of Colleagues

Idealist
- Rejects or fails to understand the security perspective
- Nursing perspective is the primary consideration
- Poorly socialized to the custody staff culture

Realist
- Acknowledges and respects the security perspective
- Nursing perspective remains the primary consideration
- Socialized to the custody staff culture

Situationalist
- Alternates between the security and the nursing perspective
- Nursing perspective is optional
- Not yet socialized to the custody staff culture

Acceptor
- Accepts the security perspective
- Minimally acknowledges the nursing perspective
- Socialized to the custody staff culture

Identifier
- Extreme acceptance of and identification with the security perspective
- Considers nursing perspective not applicable in a jail environment
- Well socialized to custody staff culture

What is the optimum work style? The researchers do not clearly note the best work style and suggest that more research is needed. The Realist style, however, seems most beneficial as this nurse is able to maintain a professional nursing perspective while understanding the perspective of correctional officers and socializing to the correctional culture. This provides an atmosphere of respect and understanding among peers while allowing for professional nursing practice.

Chapter 5: Same Dorothy, Though

Yes, as different as nursing is inside the security perimeter, being a nurse does not change. Dorothy did not stop being a young girl from Kansas when she started down the Yellow Brick Road to find her way back home. In fact, it was in this journey that she truly found herself. Practicing as a nurse in the correctional setting can be, at first, unsettling, but can lead to a true understanding of who you are as a nurse and how you make a difference for your patients.

Stripped of the many supports that are standard in traditional settings, such as a nursing administration or a team of like-minded staff members, many correctional nurses must carve their own path to professional practice behind bars. This is when it is most important to understand the boundaries of your license and the Nurse Practice Act for your state or jurisdiction (here is a handy directory of State NPAs). This is also when an understanding of the professional Code of Ethics for Nurses is important. The principles that guide professional practice such as patient autonomy, human dignity, and patient-centered care, are challenged every day in a correctional setting.

For many nurses, this is the first time they have been confronted with defining their own practice boundaries or needing to speak out when a request is made that is beyond their scope of practice or is unethical. Here are some recommendations to help you remain true to your professional licensure and ethical responsibilities.

- **Know your role and responsibilities**. Don't wait for a situation to arise that seems wrong to you. Review your Nurse Practice Act and how it practically applies to your correctional nursing position. For example, if you are a licensed practical/vocational nurse (LPN/LVN), are you able to assess and determine interventions for a patient condition? If not, do not accept a sick call assignment.

- **Know your job description, policies and procedures.** As with your professional role and responsibilities, know your role and responsibilities to your employer. Determine, before a situation happens, if there are any elements of these documents that don't seem appropriate to your licensure or ethical responsibilities.

- **Talk to your supervisor.** If you have concerns about what you are being asked to do, follow the chain of command and address the issues with your supervisor. Ask about a mechanism for refusing assignments that are not consistent with the Nurse Practice Act. Always work toward a positive resolution to the issue.

- **Prepare a good response to an officer request.** Have a well-thought-out response for when you are asked by an officer or security administrator to perform a function that is outside your professional or ethical boundaries. Remember, these folks may not know they are asking you to do something unlawful or unethical. Give them the benefit of the doubt. Here is an example to get you started thinking about how you can respond respectfully and collegially: "I'd really like to help you out with this issue, but what you are asking me to do is beyond what my nursing license allows (or is not considered ethical for a nurse to do). Let's see if we can come up with a solution that works for all of us."

All of the recommendations above address the issue of being asked to work outside the boundaries of professional nursing practice, but there is another concern that you need to be ever alert for – leaving your nursing license at the door when you walk in. Only you can maintain that mental attitude of who you are as a nurse and what your goals are for professional practice. The definition of correctional nursing found in the ANA's Correctional Nursing Scope and Standards of Practice is a good place to start for creating your own mission statement for your work as a correctional nurse:

> *Correctional nursing is the protection, promotion, and optimization of health and abilities, prevention of illness and injury, alleviation of suffering through the diagnosis and treatment of human response, advocacy, and delivery of health care to individuals, families, communities, and populations under the jurisdiction of the criminal justice system.*

Using this definition as a guide, you can be reminded of what you do, how you do it and where you are practicing.

What I Do

- Protect and promote health
- Prevent illness and injury
- Alleviate suffering

How I Do It

- Through the nursing process
- By being a patient advocate

Chapter 5: Same Dorothy, Though

Where I Do It

- In the criminal justice system

Dorothy was always Dorothy in the Land of Oz and we must remain professional nurses while practicing in the criminal justice system. By doing so, we make a difference in the lives of a needy patient population and, in many ways, help humanize the incarceration experience.

SECTION II

If I Only Had a Brain
Correctional Nurse Knowledge

"I haven't got a brain... only straw." – The Scarecrow

Dorothy's first companion on the Yellow Brick Road was the Scarecrow. He decided to accompany her to see the Wizard and obtain a brain to replace the straw in his head. It is easy to feel like you have a head full of straw when first encountering the correctional nursing field. There is so much that is new to learn. This section guides you through the most important components of the knowledge needed to deliver nursing care in a jail or prison.

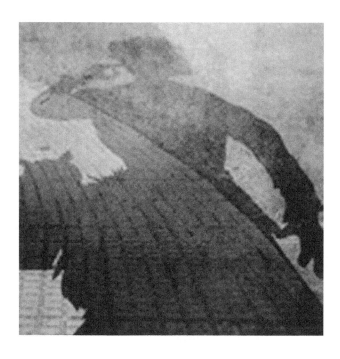

Chapter 6: Health Care Processes

Healthcare is provided in secure settings through several standard processes. These processes ensure that necessary care is consistently delivered and that patients have access to health care when they think they need it. Health care begins upon entry into the facility through an intake assessment and continues throughout confinement. Acute needs are handled through the sick call process while chronic diseases are managed through chronic care clinics. Medical and mental health emergency care is also managed. Often called man-down situations, health care staff can be called to any area of the facility to assess and treat a health emergency. Continuing treatment and monitoring takes place in an infirmary or observation area. Some facilities may have a long-term care program within the infirmary or an entire facility may be designated for care of those inmates with long-term or hospice needs.

Intake Screening and Health Assessment

Intake screening is the primary process used to determine the immediate and ongoing health needs of inmates coming into the correctional system.

Purpose

There are four main purposes of an intake screening.

Emergency. The first purpose is to identify any impending health care emergencies. For example, there may have been a traumatic arrest process that created injuries that need attention.

Urgent Care. Urgent health needs are also a concern. An entering inmate may have a communicable condition that needs immediate treatment or they may be an insulin-dependent diabetic without their medication for many hours during the arrest process.

Health Review. During an intake screening, a review of medical conditions may lead to the registration of the person in various chronic care clinics such as hypertension management or being placed on the schedule for prenatal visits.

Referral. The intake screening can also lead to referral for additional evaluations such as a mental health evaluation for suicide potential.

Phases

There are three primary phases of entry into the health care system in a correctional setting. These phases may be accomplished in various ways depending on the physical and organizational set up of the facility.

Phase I: Medical Clearance. Medical Clearance takes place first and involves an evaluation of emergent medical or psychiatric needs that must be addressed before entry into the facility. Primarily, this involves consciousness, bleeding, or extensive trauma. This determination is made before accepting the individual for booking. Those with immediate need for emergency treatment are sent to a hospital.

Phase II: Receiving Screening. If accepted through the medical clearance, the next two phases can be done separately or together. The receiving screening process can be preliminary to a later full assessment or combined with a full assessment. The nature of intake screening causes it to be the more risky part of the health care intake and should be done as soon as possible in the booking process to determine urgent and emergent health needs. Screening involves brief inquiry into key health issues and observations of physical appearance.

Key Health Questions during a Receiving Screening

- Current and past illnesses, health conditions, or special health requirements such as dietary needs
- Past serious infectious diseases
- Recent communicable illness symptoms like chronic cough, fever, loss of appetite, or night sweats
- Past or current mental illness, including hospitalizations
- History of or current suicidal ideation
- Dental problems
- Allergies
- Legal and illegal drug use
- Drug withdrawal symptoms
- Current or recent pregnancy
- Key screening observations
- Appearance of illness (sweating, tremors, anxiety, disheveled)
- Behavior (disorderly, appropriate, insensible)

- State of consciousness (alert, responsive, lethargic)
- Ease of movement (body deformities, gait, balance)
- Breathing (cough, hyperventilation)
- Skin (rashes, jaundice, bruises, tattoos, needle marks or indication of drug use)

Phase III: Health Assessment. Finally, the initial health assessment can take place along with the receiving screening or can take place later in the process. Accreditation standards require an initial health assessment as soon as possible but within seven days of prison admission and within 14 days of a jail admission. This initial assessment adds a physical exam to the receiving screening information and provides a more complete picture of the individual's health status and health needs.

Risks at Intake

The nature of the inmate population in general and the characteristics of your particular population lead to some special risk areas in the intake screening and assessment process. It is important to be aware of these risk areas and put into place the safeguards that will catch these conditions and triage patients into appropriate treatment processes.

Self-Harm. Suicide is a significant correctional health care issue that should be addressed from intake onward in the incarceration timeline. Suicide rates in county jails have dropped over the last few decades but are still more than three times higher than in the general public. Screening for suicide potential, then, is an important function of the intake screening process. There are reasons individuals may wish to be less than truthful in sharing their past suicide history or their current ideations. So, sensitivity is needed when asking about suicide at intake.

Drugs and Alcohol. More than 80% of our patients are substance involved – either alcohol or illegal drugs. Potential for alcohol or drug withdrawal is therefore a major concern in the initial health screening. Obtaining truthful information can be challenging and the screener should use caution in determining the need for withdrawal monitoring.

Prescription Medications. A third area of concern in the intake screening process is medication that the person may be currently taking. Determining the exact medication and dosage can be difficult. Inmates can arrive with a bottle of mixed medications or just a verbal list of general names like 'my pressure pill' and 'my sugar pill'. Getting accurate information about these medications and validating information with the prescriber can be a challenge.

Chronic Care Clinics

Once evaluated for immediate and continuing health care needs during intake, many in the inmate patient population will require ongoing assessment and treatment of chronic conditions. This takes place through the chronic care clinic process.

The inmate patient population is disproportionately black and low-income. Ethnic minorities from poor backgrounds report higher prevalence of chronic diseases. Factors contributing to chronic disease such as substance abuse, excessive tobacco and alcohol, poor diets and limited medical care prior to incarceration, are also present. Longer sentences have increased the number of older inmates in the criminal justice system. The incarcerated patient population has need of regular attention to chronic diseases. The chronic care clinic process reduces the frequency and severity of symptoms, prevents disease progression and complications, and encourages improved functioning.

Common Chronic Disease Services

- Asthma
- Diabetes
- High Blood Cholesterol
- HIV
- Hypertension
- Seizure Disorder
- Tuberculosis
- Major Mental Illness

The frequency of clinic visits is determined by the nature of the condition and the needs of the individual patient. Many facilities set a standard for visit frequency at every 90 days with more frequent visits if the condition is unstable, treatments are being adjusted, or diagnostic testing has been ordered and needs more frequent review.

The chronic care visit is an ideal time for patient teaching and reinforcement. Every interaction with a patient is an opportunity to inform, build rapport, and promote good health.

Chronic care visits may be handled in conjunction with other visits to the health care unit, such as sick call. Coordination of the chronic care process with security administration improves efficiency and reduces manpower needs.

Chapter 6: Health Care Processes

Finding Clinical Guidelines

Correctional practitioners are required to care for the inmate patient population equivalent to those in the community. Following nationally recognized guidelines reduces the risk of legal liability for negligent care. Here is a quick-start list of resources for guidelines that work well in a correctional setting.

Community Sources

- Agency for Healthcare Research and Quality
- National Heart, Lung, and Blood Institute
- National Institutes of Health AIDS*info* Web site
- National Institute for Health and Care Excellence (NICE)
- American Diabetes Association
- The American College of Rheumatology (ACR)

Corrections-Specific Sources

- Federal Bureau of Prisons (FBOP) Clinical Practice Guidelines
- National Commission on Correctional Health Care (NCCHC) Guidelines for Disease Management

Sick Call

The sick call process was developed to allow access to care for acute non-emergent conditions, similar to a doctor's office visit. Due to limitations on movement and the inability to seek out care and treatment as they would in the free world, inmates must have a way to make known a need for evaluation and treatment by a health care professional. Most correctional facilities have a nurse sick call and provider sick call appointment process with the patient first seeing the nurse for triage and initial evaluation of symptoms.

Inmates should be instructed about how to access health care early in the incarceration process. In jails, this might occur during the health screening. In prisons, this could also happen during the facility orientation program. Reinforcement of access, such as signs and forms, should be available in the housing units.

The plan for non-emergency access to medical, dental, and mental health services should allow an inmate to refer him or herself for preliminary evaluation. Many facilities use a written request process, but some settings now use a verbal voicemail or a kiosk system for requests. Whatever system is used, it should be confidential and only accessible by health care staff. In the simple paper request system, a locked dropbox is often available on every housing unit. Inmates obtain request slips from the housing officer, complete the information and submit to the dropbox where health care staff pick up requests on daily rounds.

Access to care should be timely to be able to address health conditions before they progress or to limit prolonged discomfort. Generally, a reasonable amount of time would result in resolution of a sick call request within 24 – 72 hours; however, all requests should be reviewed by a qualified health professional upon receipt to ensure urgent requests are prioritized for immediate evaluation. In some medium and minimum security settings, sick call is managed without written requests through standard open hours when inmates can request a pass to be seen in the sick call clinic.

Sick call requests are triaged based on indication of urgent need and type of request. For example, a request about severe abdominal pain might be triaged for immediate evaluation by a nurse and then placed for a follow-up visit with the provider; while a request indicating itchy feet might be placed on the nurse sick call schedule for the next available opening.

Written medically-approved nursing protocols guide acute care decision-making during a nursing sick call visit. Protocols identify the types of assessments that should be made for various presenting symptoms and then identify treatment options once assessment findings verify a diagnosis. For nurses, the treatment options can include over-the-counter remedies, instruction on self-care, patient education, and scheduling a follow-up visit with a provider for prescriptive treatment or further evaluation. Only in special situations, such as emergencies, are nurses able to administer prescription medications through protocols – and only within licensure standards until a provider is contacted for orders.

Infirmary Care

Many correctional facilities have infirmary units with cells grouped for immediate access by health care staff. These areas are created to accommodate patients needing daily monitoring, medication, therapy and assistance at a skilled nursing level but not at the level of a hospital. Due to the secure nature of the housing units, these patients require care that cannot be managed safely in the housing areas due to unsafe conditions such as needles or medical equipment that could serve as weapons.

Infirmary patients require an active nursing presence and should be within sight or hearing of a care provider at all times. Admission and discharge orders should be

Chapter 6: Health Care Processes

written by a provider. Examples of conditions that might require infirmary admission are:

- Continuous and intermittent IV therapy
- Complex wound management
- Need for equipment unsafe in the general population, such as feeding pumps or crutches
- Infectious disease isolation, such as suspected tuberculosis or chicken pox
- Continuous observation needs, such as potential concussion or post-operative release from hospital

In addition to sub-acute care situations, infirmaries can also be used to handle long-term care needs of inmates such as spinal cord injury or hospice care.

Infirmaries should have security officers assigned to the area for personal safety purposes. Health care staff should be sure that officers are nearby and aware when entering infirmary cells to assess the patient or administer medications and treatments.

Emergency Response

Medical or mental health emergencies can happen in any location within a correctional facility. Health care staff must be ready to manage these emergencies. This means first aid and gaining access to appropriate follow-up evaluation and treatment.

When responding to an emergency outside the health care unit, safety of self, other staff, and other inmates comes first. Officers will clear the area of safety threats before allowing health care staff to evaluate the patient. Without this precaution, many more individuals than the one with the health emergency could be in jeopardy. Once given clearance, provide initial treatment according to standard emergency and first aid protocols.

Emergency Medical Service response can be delayed by the various security processes for facility entry and by the actual location of the event within the facility. Ongoing stabilization of the patient, then, can be prolonged. If officers have been trained in CPR and First Aid, they can help in the team effort while awaiting outside assistance. In an unwitnessed situation, always consider a neck injury. Stabilize the patient's neck manually and then with a collar until the C-spine has been cleared.

The first health care professional at the scene is in charge until replaced by another of equal or higher qualification to manage the emergency. Under no circumstance should an emergency scene be left, even to obtain needed supplies, unless relieved by another equally qualified health professional. Instead, delegate equipment retrieval to another individual on the scene such as a security officer.

Medication Administration

The secure nature of the correctional setting, along with the dispersed nature of health care delivery, has led to several unique processes for medication administration. Faulty management of the processes, poor interaction among health care and officer staff, and inappropriate use of the medication system by the patient population lead to increased risk in the system of care. Here is an overview of several common ways that medications are delivered in a secure setting, with safety tips for each method.

Medication Line (Pill Line)

The primary means of administering scheduled medication to the incarcerated patient population is through a medication line-up. In this process, patients needing medication are queued at a dispersion point. Depending on facility layout or organizational culture, a medication line can be centralized or decentralized.

Centralized Medication Line. A centralized process has patients come to a central location, often a pill window, where a nurse is stationed with a medication cart. The pill window may be within the health care unit or may be in a central location such as a room near the inmate dining room or other general access area. The centralized medication line in the health care unit provides for the least risky process as the nurse has access to all the resources of the health care unit, including other staff members and the medical record, when needed.

Decentralized Medication Line. In this process, the medication line comes to the housing unit. A nurse transports the medication cart from unit to unit and patients line up for medications. The location in the housing unit might be next to the officer desk or from a small room attached to the unit. The decentralized medication line has increased risk over the centralized options as the nurse is isolated from health care unit resources and other staff. The medication cart must be carefully prepared to provide access to commonly needed items. Unexpected requests, miscommunications, or missing items require notation and attention on return to the health care unit.

Safety Tips for Medication Line. Direct observation therapy medication administration has great potential for error and patient safety concerns. The pressure to work quickly and finish the line on time is intense, yet correctional nurses are accountable to follow all standard safety practices in this situation. Here are some safety tips for this form of medication administration.

Chapter 6: Health Care Processes

- *Patient Identification* – Use two forms of identification. Having the inmate state their name and show an ID number is a common practice. ID cards should have a picture, if possible. Inmates may exchange cards and use the name of another to obtain valuable medications. Some facilities require birth dates.

- *Oral Check* – Be sure someone, preferably an officer, is checking that the medication is swallowed. Inmates may 'cheek' medication for use for other purposes such as self-harm or barter on the prison black market.

- *MAR System* – Set up an efficient system for finding the patient in the medication administration record (MAR). Many facilities keep the MAR in last name order. Some also divide MAR's by housing unit. For example, one cart may go to Units A & B and another to Units C & D.

- *Medication System* – Keep the patient medication cards organized. All medication cards should have the patient name and ID affixed. Keep the patient's entire medication supply together, and preferably in alphabetical order by medication. It helps if someone is responsible for keeping order, such as a pharmacy tech (if you have that luxury).

- *Discontinued Medications* – Get rid of discontinued medication to avoid confusion and error. Keep discontinued medications off the cart or out of the administration area.

- *Calculations* – If a calculation is needed to administer the correct dose, write a double-checked calculation on the MAR. For example, 1.5 tabs = 75mg.

- *Minimize Strength Options* – A variety of strengths of a single medication in stock can lead to dose errors in administration. Keep choices to a minimum.

- *Similar Names* – Drugs that look alike or sound alike should be separated and clearly labeled with the name. Some units underline the differences in the name to emphasize the differences for staff when selecting medication for administration.

- *Documenting Administration* – Document in the MAR at the time of administration – not before pill line or after returning to the health care unit. Before administration, you don't know if the patient will show for pill line or if they might refuse the medication. After pill line, you can't rely on memory or may get tied up with emergencies and miss documenting altogether.

- *Using Other Patient's Medications* – In a resource-scarce environment like a correctional facility, it is tempting to overstep bounds in order to provide needed medications to patients. Do not give medications ordered for one patient to another patient, even if it is the same medication. This is faulty nursing practice and can even be considered illegal, as taking this action moves the function from medication administration to medication dispensing.

No Shows to Pill Line. Patients not showing up for the pill line can be a problem in some facilities. Although tracking down patients who do not show up for their medications can be time-consuming, it is important for both the therapeutic and legal nature of medication administration. A consistent documentation process should be in place to show that every effort was made to administer ordered medication to the intended patient. Because access to care is a legal concern for incarcerated patients, without proper documentation it could be construed that the patient was intentionally denied their medication.

In many settings, a patient who does not show for two consecutive pill lines is scheduled for an appointment with the prescriber to discuss treatment refusal. Some settings also require patients to come to the medication cart and sign a refusal slip. In all cases, a tracking system must be in place to confirm that the patient had access to the medication that was ordered for them.

Cell-side Medication Delivery

When patients are unable to leave their cell, medication must be delivered directly to the cell. Patients may be confined due to their classification, administrative segregation, a facility lock-down, or other safety concern. This process usually requires pre-packaging of medication, although some facilities are arranged so that there is opportunity to roll the medication cart from cell to cell. Using the medication cart with MAR is the optimum method for cell-side medication delivery. Pre-packaging medication administration is more risky than medication line administration as the preparation and administration of medication is distanced by time and location.

Pre-packaged/Pre-poured Medication. Although pre-packaging or pre-pouring medication is a risky practice, it is a fact of life in some correctional settings due to security processes and a physical layout that does not allow the movement of a medication cart to the administration area – often a housing unit. When it is necessary to pre-pour medications, patient doses are packaged in small envelopes in the medication room and then transported and directly delivered to the patient. Pre-packaging medications and then transporting them to the patient adds an extra layer of complexity to the process and should be done only when necessary and with added caution.

Safety Tips for Pre-packaged Medication Administration. Here are some tips for pre-packaged medication administration to reduce the risk of error.

- The person preparing the medication should also administer it. Administration should come directly after packaging to reduce errors of distraction or memory.

- The packaging container (often a small envelope) needs to be sealed and labeled with basic identifying information such as patient name, date of birth, medication name, dose, frequency, and any hold parameters.

- Be prepared to identify and address any challenge to the medication by the patient. For example, if the patient challenges the accuracy of a dose given to them, how will you respond?

- Do not pre-sign the MAR before administering the medication dose. The error margin is great. A medication may be held or refused.

- Obtaining an area roster before medication preparation can omit those discharged or not available for med pass and reduce the volume and amount of medications pre-poured but not administered.

Keep-On-Person/Self-Administered Medication

Keep on Person (KOP) medication administration is a common practice in many jails and prisons. This process allows inmates to keep a quantity of medications (usually 30 days) with them and self-administer according to the directions provided. Since most adults in the community self-administer prescription and over-the-counter medication, this seems a prudent practice. There are, however, several concerns that need to be addressed to successfully manage a KOP process.

Medications, like any material item, can be a commodity on the prison black market. Pills can be used for both intended and unintended purposes. In an environment of scarcity, community members will creatively use whatever is available to barter or gain status in the group.

Each facility determines which medications are safe for inmates to carry with them based on the population characteristics and past experience. The need for consistent administration may also be taken into account when determining self-administration medication classes. For example, tuberculosis medication administration is rarely left to the discretion of the patient as consistent dosing over a long period of time is necessary for maximum effect. Another class of medications often eliminated from KOP lists is psychotropic medications. Patient adherence to daily psychotropic medication dosing can be a challenge even in the general community. In addition, many psychotropic medications can be abused. Vulnerable inmates with desirable medications on their person can become prey to stronger and more powerful inmates and gangs.

Safety Tips for Self-Administered Medications. Here are some tips for a safe and effective KOP medication program.

- There should be a consistent process for distributing and reordering KOP medications. Be sure inmates understand the system and their responsibilities. Many medical units ask that inmates show up at a treatment or pill line to reorder medications when there are about 10 doses left. This allows time for order filling.

- Incorporate KOP medication into the Medication Administration Record (MAR) process. All medications provided to the patient should be documented in a single place to assist in communication among care providers and decrease confusion in the treatment plan.

- Be sure every medication card has the patient's name and ID, as well as medication and prescription information. During cell sweeps, medications will be confiscated if not in the possession of the person whose name is on the card.

- Security staff should be able to confirm the rightful owner of any medication found in the general prison population.

- A regular spot-check process for patient compliance with self-administered medications is helpful. Randomly check medication cards in mid-cycle to determine proper use. For example, twice a week, a number of inmates with KOP medications could be called to report to the medical unit with all medication cards. Nurses can use this time to validate proper use and reinforce patient teaching.

Involving the patient in administering their own medications can improve patient safety and assist with developing independent health habits. Patient education on drug and food interactions is important, as is information about medication effects and side effects. Confirm that the patient understands conditions that require medical attention and the process for obtaining more medication when the supply is dwindling.

Infirmary Medication Delivery

Some patients are confined to cells within a health care unit for medical needs that cannot be managed in the general population. While general population medications are primarily oral and topical, infirmary medications can include intravenous and injectable medications. Needle use is risky in housing areas. Medications infrequently used can be required in the infirmary setting, adding to administration risk.

Emergency Medication Delivery

Correctional health care staff respond to medical emergencies (man-down) throughout the compound. A medication emergency kit is transported to the scene and can include various emergency preparations such as Epinephrine, Benedryl, cardiac medications, Narcan, and glucose.

Med Packs and Sick Call Dosing

Medications are also delivered to patients during direct care visits with the nurse or provider. In the case of nursing sick call, over-the-counter medications may be administered for minor conditions such as athlete's foot, seasonal allergy, or indigestion. Nursing sick call may be provided at a time and location disconnected from the medical record or medication administration record. Thus, these additional medications may not get documented into the patient's medical history; even though over-the-counter medications also have potential to interact with or affect the action of prescription medications. Likewise, prescription medications of short duration may be offered to patients during the course of provider sick call. Documentation of this administration in the medical record, particularly in the MAR, is important for the overall management of the patient's health.

- If providers give out medications during sick call, sometimes called 'Provider Packs', the medication cards should have the inmate's name and ID written on them by the provider along with date and signature.

- In like fashion, non-prescription or over-the-counter medication distributed by nurses during sick call should be labeled for the individual inmate with date and nurse signature.

Officer Medication Delivery

State regulation varies as to how medication may be delivered such that an officer may be able to deliver medication to inmates that has been prepared by a nurse for distribution. This method is more frequent in settings with reduced health care staffing, such as small local jails. The medical authority may treat this process as delivering medication for patient self-administration. This method of medication administration, then, is of highest risk as it combines issues of both KOP and pre-packaging of medication. Officer medication delivery adds an additional risk as the medication is given to the patient by someone other than the nurse who prepared it. There is no certainty that the patient actually took the medication unless the officer watches. Communication of missed doses or refusals can be difficult. In additions, officers must be thoroughly trained for medication delivery and regularly monitored for correct practices. In this era of complex medication regimens and high potential for error, officer medication delivery is not recommended as a safe process.

Special Issues When Administering Medications in Corrections

The correctional health care setting has several special safety issues when administering medications. Let's take a look at some tips for reducing errors in these situations.

The Medication Timing Challenge. The timing of medication administration is often determined by the security schedule. Yet a system for consistently providing ordered medication is needed to assure therapeutic response. The professional standard is for medication to be administered within an hour of the scheduled dose. The correctional environment can be unpredictable and medication administration can come to a screeching halt when security needs to 'lock down' movement for a safety concern.

For those time periods where medications cannot be safely administered one hour before or after the time designated or facility med pass protocol, an alternative plan must be in place to address life-threatening medication regimens. Collaboration between security and health care is crucial to make arrangements for time-sensitive medications or where omissions could place a patient in jeopardy. Many medications are specifically timed due to the action or effects intended by their use. For example, some medication should be taken on an empty stomach and others taken with food for best absorption.

Staff Safety. Medication management processes can be a source of potential staff injury. Slack processes can lead to inappropriate patient access to medications through diversion by staff or hoarding by patients. This can lead to increased violence, overdose and suicide attempts. Here are important steps to ensure medication security.

- Keeping all medication in a locked area and narcotics under double lock (for example, a locked cabinet in a locked room).
- Attending medication at all times when they are outside the locked medication room.
- Reducing the number of staff who have access to medication room keys.
- Maintaining a security escort when in possession of medications in an inmate area.
- Heightened awareness when patients are in a patient care area with access to medications such as medication pass or sick call.

Chapter 6: Health Care Processes

Staff safety during the medication administration process is an important concern in corrections, as well. Patients can become volatile when medication requests are declined. Because drug-seeking behaviors may be present, staff should be wary to maintain protocol and only administer verifiable ordered medications. A casual nature in administering medication can encourage a culture of manipulation and places staff at risk for blackmail and professional ruin.

Where the cart is placed is a component of safety. For example, can the cart be shoved back at you if a patient becomes unruly? Where is the security officer standing in relation to the cart? Is the patient an arm's length away so that items can't be grabbed and used as a weapon?

Staff safety can also be compromised by an employee's own medication practices. Prescribed and therapeutic medications taken by staff members may impair decision-making. A discussion with the unit manager and a temporary altered assignment may be necessary while taking medications with these potential side effects.

Verbal and Telephone Orders. Orders communicated verbally are common in all clinical settings with estimates as high as 20% of all inpatient ordering. However, verbal or telephone orders are probably more frequently used in correctional settings than traditional settings as prescribers are often less accessible in our secure environment.

The most common verbal order errors involve misinterpretation of the dose or the medication name. Some common examples include misinterpreting the number fifteen (15) as being fifty (50) and the number two (2) as being ten (10). Besides dosage confusion, sound-alike medications have also caused errors. Examples here include mistaking azithromycin for erythromycin and klonopin for clonidine.

To reduce the chance for error, all verbal orders should be read back to the prescriber before implementation. The read-back process requires the staff member who receives a verbal order to read-back the order information and obtain affirmation from the prescriber that the information is accurate. The read-back process includes the following components.

- The receiving staff member writes down the order as it is spoken by the prescriber.

- The receiving staff member repeats the order back to the prescriber – reading directly from the written dictation.

- To reduce sound-alike errors in medication and dosage, the reader spells out the medication name and dosage amount, for example, t-w-o – 2 mg.

- A verbal affirmation is obtained from the prescriber before initiating the order.
- A second staff member qualified to accept verbal orders listens in on highly risky communications such as insulin, anticoagulants, and narcotics.

The high risk of error with verbal orders requires limits on use. Here are some standard limits placed on verbal orders that should be considered in our setting.

- Limit verbal orders to urgent patient care needs and not as a routine practice or for convenience purposes.
- Limit the number of staff who can take verbal orders.
- Limit the type of medication that can be ordered to formulary medications that are more likely to be familiar to staff members.
- Do not use verbal orders for complex medication schemes such as chemotherapy.

Summary

Standard correctional health care processes have been developed over time to accommodate the primary care delivery needs in criminal justice settings. An understanding of these processes along with key areas for patient and staff safety concern will help you to navigate the system and delivery nursing care.

Chapter 7: High Risk Issues

The particulars of the incarcerated patient population and the characteristics of the secure environment of care lead to increased health care activity involving several nursing concerns. Three over-arching concerns should be top-of-mind for nurses working behind bars: suicide and self-injury, substance withdrawal, and infectious disease. These three issues make up a large portion of the legal cases involving correctional health care.

Suicide

Incarceration is a traumatic and stressful life experience that can lead to mental decline and experiences of extreme loss. This, combined with high rates of mental illness in the patient community, results in high risk for patient self-harm or suicide attempts. Suicide rates in corrections are much higher than the general public, with the highest rates in jail settings. Suicides are most common in smaller jails.

Suicide Awareness through the Continuum

The majority of suicide attempts in the criminal justice system take place within the first days behind bars; therefore, the early period of incarceration is very important for observation. However, suicide attempts can be triggered by other life-affecting events. Here are a few high-risk periods.

- New legal problems, such as new charges, additional sentences, institutional proceedings, or denial of parole
- Receipt of bad news regarding self or family, such as serious illness, loss of a loved one, or divorce proceedings
- Suffering humiliation, such as a sexual assault
- Even pending release after long incarceration can trigger a suicide attempt

Therefore, be vigilant for any indication that a patient's mental status is deteriorating, as this can lead to a self-harming action. Remain alert for suicide potential with all patients. This can be challenging, especially at the mid and final points of the inmate's sentencing when routine is established and attention shifts to other concerns.

Intake screening is a primary place to assess for suicide potential. Most settings will include a series of questions about suicide during entry into the facility. Suicide attempts are more likely in individuals who have attempted suicide in the past, have family members who have committed suicide or if they have witnessed a suicide in the past. Therefore the following questions may be a part of intake screening.

- Past history of suicide attempts or self-injury behaviors
- Family suicide history
- Current suicide ideation
- Realistic plan to commit suicide
- Command hallucinations to kill self

If entering inmates indicate any of these signs of suicide potential, they should be monitored and evaluated further by mental health staff. Often the intake nurse is responsible to initiate monitoring and evaluation processes.

Suicide Prevention Interventions

Patients who show suicide potential are placed into a monitored situation for their safety. Two levels of monitoring are standard in correctional settings.

- **Constant Observation**. Actively suicidal inmates are placed on constant observation. A staff member is continually present and observing the patient for suicide attempt.

- **Close Watch**. Potentially suicidal inmates are placed on close watch. They are monitored on an irregular schedule with no more than 15 minutes between checks.

Placing a patient on suicide precautions is often performed by nurses based on the screening process; however, removal from suicide precautions should be limited to licensed mental health professionals.

Responding to a Hanging Suicide Attempt

Although the incarcerated patient population can attempt suicide through a number of means, hanging is the most common form of successful suicide in corrections. The actions taken in the first few minutes after a discovered hanging can be the difference between a hospital transfer and an in-custody death. Here are some tips for effectively responding to a hanging.

- The major factors leading to a hanging fatality are height of the drop during hanging and the suspension of the body (full or partial). Most hangings in corrections take place in the housing area (primarily the inmate cell) which leaves little chance for a full body suspension and great height. This results in good chances of survival with early intervention. Even if the victim is found to be lifeless, aggressive intervention with CPR and emergency medical transport is warranted.

- A significant percentage of hanging victims will have spinal fracture, therefore spine immobilization and jaw thrust maneuvers should be taken into account at the scene.

- Easy access to a rescue tool, such as a seatbelt release device, is needed to quickly lower the person to the floor for emergency resuscitation intervention. This tool may be provided in the emergency response bag or available from custody officers.

There have been reports of medical staff being delayed from attending to a hanging victim while crime scene investigation takes place. Minutes are precious in emergency treatment and can make a difference in ultimate survival. Cut down the victim and initiate emergency medical intervention as soon as the scene has been secured. Saving a person's life trumps all need for determining criminality. Nurses must advocate for immediate patient treatment in this situation. Even better, pre-empt an emergency situation like this by determining whether the facility has such a policy or process before a hanging event.

Self-Injury

Self-injury behavior is a misunderstood phenomenon that is quite prevalent in the inmate population. An estimated 2 – 4% of the general prison population engage in the activity. The most common forms of self-injury in the correctional setting are cutting, inserting or swallowing objects, head banging, and opening old wounds. Working in corrections, you will definitely be confronted with inmates who have self inflicted bleeding, bruising and burning damage.

Although self-injury may, at first, appear to be a desire for attention or a response to boredom, some mental health experts are finding the behavior to be motivated by a 'coping deficit' when dealing with feelings of depression or powerlessness. Many who self-injure have a history of childhood physical or sexual abuse. Children experiencing repeated abuse often cope by dissociation from the physical and psychological pain. This same dissociation from pain is seen in some who self-injure. Self-injury may act to release endorphins that calm the individual, thereby relieving stress for a time.

No matter the cause of the behavior, those who self-injure will need both medical and mental health attention. A concerted, multi-disciplinary response is needed. Interventions may include intensive therapy, group sessions, and careful treatment planning. A collaboration of custody and treatment efforts is a better answer to managing this condition.

Substance Withdrawal

The majority of the incarcerated population meets clinical standards for alcohol and drug abuse or addiction. Entry into the criminal justice system means the elimination of access to substances that may be needed for physical and mental stability. Ensuing withdrawal can cause instability, suffering, and death. Alcohol withdrawal has the highest mortality rate, but withdrawal from depressant drugs and opiates can also be life-threatening.

Like suicide and self-injuries, discussed earlier, substance withdrawal should be evaluated on intake through a standard screening process. Screening should include the type, amount, frequency, duration of use, and history of past withdrawal symptoms. This information can help determine the level of withdrawal monitoring and intervention needed during the incarceration process.

Alcohol Withdrawal

Withdrawal from alcohol causes increased excitability in the nervous system leading to nausea, vomiting, sweating, shakiness, agitation and anxiety. A medical emergency can develop when withdrawal leads to delirium tremens (DT's) involving hallucinations, confusion, disorientation, and generalized seizures. Autonomic hyper-reactivity can progress to hypertension, tachycardia, hyperthermia, rapid breathing, and tremors.

Although the mild to moderate withdrawal symptoms will peak and wane in the first 2 days, DT's occur around 48 – 72 hours after the last drink. Untreated DT's can lead to cardiovascular collapse. Here are the primary areas of alcohol withdrawal assessment and management.

Assessment and Monitoring. The most tested assessment tool for the identification of persons at risk for alcohol withdrawal is the Clinical Institute Withdrawal Assessment of Alcohol Scale (CIWA-AR). It uses a numbering system to objectively determine severity of withdrawal and can be used over time to document the course of alcohol withdrawal for an individual inmate. Twice daily CIWA-AR assessment is recommended for those determined to be vulnerable.

Hydration. High on the list of non-pharmacologic interventions for alcohol withdrawal is hydration. Alcoholics are often dehydrated, which increases nervous system excitability. Encourage withdrawing inmates to increase fluids by mouth. Some facilities provide electrolyte replacement fluids, such as Gatorade or other sports drink to withdrawing inmates, as alcohol-dependent individuals are often electrolyte depleted.

Nutrition. The chronic drinker is also likely to be glycogen-depleted and malnourished. These conditions enhance alcohol withdrawal symptoms. Get these folks into the meal system pronto. Encourage nutritious eating to replace these stores. Good choices to have available are milk, sandwiches and peanut butter crackers.

Medication. Reducing nervous system excitability will decrease chances of life-threatening DT's. Providing a short-term (5-day) taper of Librium, Valium or other barbiturate will decrease the chances for respiratory and cardiovascular collapse. Of course, a physician order is needed for this intervention. Many settings have a standard protocol for barbiturate treatment with stock medication available for immediate initiation.

Hospitalization. If you are unable to forestall seizures, hallucinations or hemodynamic instability, arrange for emergency transport to the nearest emergency room. These patients need a level of care beyond that able to be given in a correctional setting.

Drug Withdrawal

Although alcohol withdrawal can have a more deadly outcome, drug withdrawal is also an important concern in this patient population. If intake screening indicates current excessive drug use, a drug withdrawal monitoring program should be initiated. The most common drug withdrawals requiring intervention in the correctional setting are benzodiazepines such as Valium, Ativan, and Xanax, and opiates such as heroin, morphine, and oxycodone.

Benzodiazepine Withdrawal. This class of drug produces central nervous system depression and so withdrawal symptoms will include anxiety, insomnia, restlessness, agitation, and muscle tension. A rapid withdrawal from high doses of the drug can also initiate seizure activity. Many benzodiazepines are long-acting so withdrawal may last up to 5 days. If symptoms are severe, a short-acting barbiturate such as phenobarbital may be ordered to lesson severity. Otherwise, treatment is usually limited to maintaining hydration and treating nausea and diarrhea.

Opiate Withdrawal. Early opiate withdrawal symptoms can be similar to benzodiazepine withdrawal but intensify to include abdominal cramping, severe muscle ache, and sweating. A standard evaluation tool such as the Clinical Opioid Withdrawal Scale (COWS) is often used to monitor symptoms and guide treatment that can include medications to treat symptoms such as diarrhea, cramping, and anxiety.

A Word about Drug Overdose. Some inmates will find ways to obtain drugs even while incarcerated. Therefore, it is not uncommon to see drug overdoses even in those who have been behind bars for some time. Drug overdose should always be considered when the patient presents as over-sedated and hypotensive with pinpoint pupils. Narcan administration should be initiated in these situations.

Infectious Disease

Healthcare is not the primary purpose of correctional settings and our patient population has higher likelihood of infectious disease than the general public. Added to this are overcrowded conditions, delays in treatment, and rationed access to soap and water; all playing a part in increased infection transmission. The inmate patient population has high rates of all primary infection classes and can have poor personal hygiene habits. The closed environment of a correctional setting can mean the quick spread of infection among the community – both inmates and staff. Correctional nurses must be especially vigilant about infection transmission practices.

Infection Transmission Prevention

Preventing infection transmission is particularly important and particularly challenging in a correctional setting. Attention to hand hygiene, standard precautions, and infection control education is needed.

Hand Hygiene. There is nothing really new about the primary infection control action – washing your hands! Yet, with all this knowledge and all this evidence before us, hand washing frequency is abysmally below standard requirements. Correctional nurses encounter many unique barriers to increasing hand hygiene practices.

- Many areas in which clinical care is provided lack hand washing stations. Correctional facilities were not designed for health care practices.

- Soap and soap dispensers are valuable commodities and may be stolen by inmates.

- Alcohol-based hand washes burn with a clear flame and may raise concerns with custody staff.

An additional peculiarity of the correctional setting is our patient population's propensity to take advantage of available resource for their benefit. To wit, inmates have been known to drink alcohol-based hand sanitizer. Although the CDC has not officially supported alcohol-free hand sanitizers, they are growing in popularity in correctional settings.

Chapter 7: High Risk Issues

Standard Precautions. Personal protective equipment (PPE) should be available in necessary sizes and quantities at all care locations. If not, please notify management. Be sure to wear gloves when in possible contact with body fluids and change them between patients. Wearing the same gloves throughout the day is not appropriate.

Education. Education is a major infection control intervention in the correctional setting. Both custody staff and patients have misinformation or lack information about the spread of infection. The following key information points should be a regular part of interactions with patients and officers.

- How to cough into the upper arm to reduce hand transmission of virus
- Proper hand washing method and frequency
- The indications of infection that should bring an inmate to the medical unit
- The use of PPE by staff to avoid contact with blood and body fluids

Common Infection Concerns

Here are some common infection routes in the correctional setting and ways to limit transmission.

Respiratory Transmission. Respiratory infections spread quickly in housing units. Prevention of spread is key. Some facilities will keep all patients with an infectious condition in a similar housing unit to contain the spread. Flu vaccine is recommended for all patients and staff but can be of limited availability and therefore only given to the highly vulnerable elderly and chronically ill. Movement and activities within a facility may be reduced during a virus outbreak to decrease infection spread.

Other airborne infections such as varicella (chicken pox) and tuberculosis require isolation in a negative-pressure room. If your facility does not have appropriate isolation for respiratory infection, these patients will be transferred to another facility. The patient should be masked during the transport process.

Blood-borne Transmission. Needle stick injury is a major concern due to the high prevalence of blood-borne pathogens, such as HIV and Hepatitis B and C, in the incarcerated patient population. Be sure to take these sharp safety precautions:

- Sharps containers should be available in all care areas. Carrying used needles to another area for disposal will increase the chance of injury.
- Keep needle boxes less than 2/3 full. Check that there is a regular supply of empty boxes for frequent replacement. Needle stick injuries can result from trying to shove used needles into an over-full red box. In many correctional

settings, staff nurses have the responsibility for changing the needle boxes when full. On a busy unit, this may get missed.

- Do not throw other trash in the sharps box. This makes it even harder to keep available for sharps waste.
- Be sure you know how to initiate the sharp safety mechanism for the needle brand in use. If the device is unfamiliar, request a demonstration. Needle stick injury can result from incorrect initiation of a sheath protector.

Skin Transmission. Methicillin-Resistant Staphyhlococcus Aureus (MRSA) is common in the correctional setting. Any skin condition should be evaluated for this infection. The patient population is prone to transmission practices such as sharing razors, performing their own wound dressing changes and draining their own abscesses. MRSA lesions continue to be referred to as 'spider bites'. Any sick call for a 'spider bite' should be evaluated immediately for MRSA.

Botulism

Homemade alcohol is fairly common in the US prison system. Local names for prison alcohol products include hooch, pruno, juice, buck, chalk, brew and jump. The brew is most often made from fermented fruit but any food source will work. Botulism is caused by a toxin produced when a bacteria commonly found in soil is placed in an oxygen-deprived environment – like the closed containers used for DIY alcohol production. The toxin is produced during the fermentation process if no heat is applied to kill the bacteria.

It is important to act on early signs of botulism as the nerve paralysis caused by the bacterial toxin can quickly move to the respiratory muscles and lead to death. Often the first signs involve the eyes, with double vision, blurred vision, or drooping eyelids. Slurred speech and dry mouth can follow along with general muscle weakness and difficulty swallowing. Botulism can quickly progress to respiratory failure. Poisoning from botulism toxins through prison hooch can happen in a few hours or take up to 10 days to appear. A medical evaluation of symptoms is necessary to rule out other possible causes of progressing paralysis. Information about the potential of drinking homemade alcohol is important for a quick diagnosis and response. Question the patient and housing officers in a suspicious situation.

Bugs that are Really Bugs

Little critters often hitchhike into our facilities, particularly head, body, and pubic lice. Once in the door, these vermin spread by direct physical contact among close-living humans or through sharing personal items like clothing and bedding.

Chapter 7: High Risk Issues

Patients who present with itching, rashes and skin lesions should be evaluated for lice and scabies as they are fairly common in this patient population. Some facilities routinely delouse inmates entering the system but this is not recommended. Medications to treat infestation should only be ordered by a licensed prescriber after verification. Close cooperation is needed between health care and custody staff as living area, clothing, and bedding must also be treated.

Summary

The high risk issues of suicide, withdrawal, and infection are pervasive in correctional health care and need to be ever-present in the day-to-day delivery of patient care. By keeping these issues in the forefront, correctional nurses can intervene quickly to decrease patient harm and improve health for this patient population. As the primary health care provider in the criminal justice system, correctional nurses may be the first to pick up indications of pending suicide, self-harm, or withdrawal from drugs or alcohol. In addition, we play an important role in reducing the spread of infection within the closed environment.

Chapter 8: Unusual Medical Conditions

Correctional nurses encounter many of the same medical conditions seen in more traditional practice settings; and they are treated in similar ways. However, the nature of our setting and the backgrounds of our patients mean that we see an array of unusual conditions and are confronted with situations rarely seen in other settings. Whether it is rhabdomyolysis from a squatting competition, prison tattoos, or treatment after pepper spray or Tasers, correctional nurses need to know what to do. Here is a need-to-know guide to top unusual medical conditions behind bars.

Dental Issues

One of the first things you will notice entering correctional nursing practice is the importance of understanding oral assessment and dental emergencies. Most nursing schools spend little time on this topic and many nurses have not had to evaluate a patient's dental condition. Correctional nurses need to understand dental conditions as we are often the ones to determine if a patient needs to see a dentist urgently or at the next available opening.

Nurses in jails and prisons must assess for, and manage or defer, dental conditions as a part of daily practice. The inmate population, as a rule, has not had regular dental care so things can really look bad in there.

Tooth sensitivity and bleeding from gingivitis or periodontitis may not have been felt or considered by the inmate until they have withdrawn from their drugs and alcohol from the street. Once off their self-medication, dental discomforts can become a concern. Although the patient may suggest otherwise, these conditions did not appear overnight but likely were developing for some time, just not noticed. For example, poor oral hygiene can lead to such extensive tartar build-up that the teeth can chip and break, requiring removal. Gingivitis, periodontitis, and excessive tartar are not emergencies but will affect eating and require dental services.

Dental Condition Directory

Ulcers. Mouth ulcers can also develop and are not emergencies. A treatment with a simple salt water gargle is often effective. Direct the inmate to use a salt packet from the chow-line in a cup of water. Ulcers can also develop from ill-fitting dentures. In this case, a dental visit is required to evaluate need for resurfacing the dentures.

Infections. Bacterial tooth infections can irritate the tooth pulp and cause an abscess. Pain and swelling shows that infection is present. In this case, short-term antibiotic treatment is needed. Long-term treatment may require tooth removal or root canal. Root canals are not frequently done in jails. An extensive abscess may cause the face to look swollen on the affected side. It is important that the infection does not spread to the airway or eye socket. The condition should be treated before it spreads. An abscess, unlike other conditions, is going to be very tender and soft. The tooth may not appear defective. Facial trauma can result in tooth nerve death and lead to an abscess.

Dental Tori. A condition of bony growth, called dental tori, can mimic abscess but is really benign and requires no treatment. When assessing for abscess, be sure that the growth or swelling is red, soft, and tender. Dental tori are a natural color (if not irritated), firm, and non-tender.

Dental Tori

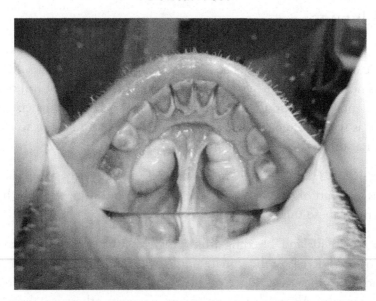

Pericoronitis. Also common in the inmate population, pericoronitis may present as an abscess but really results from an unerupted wisdom tooth. Gum tissue overgrowth can get in the way of chewing and become swollen and sore. Antibiotics will reduce swelling, if extensive. Otherwise, good oral hygiene – regular brushing, flossing and debris removal – will improve this condition.

Meth Mouth. Meth mouth is a dental condition brought on by chronic meth drug use. It involves accelerated tooth decay and loss. The intense decay can appear as an emergency requiring immediate treatment. However, this is rarely necessary. The condition is caused by the loss of saliva and increased intake of sugar. Generally the mouth does not feel painful to the patient. This decay happens quickly in 1 – 2

Chapter 8: Unusual Medical Conditions

years of meth use. Long-term meth use leads to further damage and tooth loss. Sometimes teeth break off at the gum line.

Meth Mouth

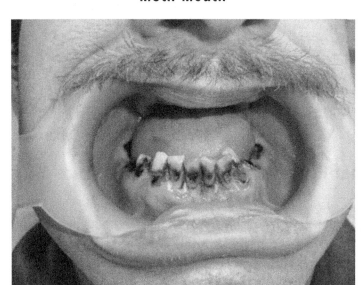

Cataloging all tooth equipment on intake is an important nursing function. This helps validate patient information later in the stay. For example, a patient might contend that a dental partial plate was taken from them during a cell sweep. This might be an expensive replacement. However, careful documentation on intake might reveal that the patient did not enter the facility with their partial. It can also important to document any broken teeth on intake. Reports from an inmate that they broke their tooth falling in their cell can be validated.

Dental Appliance Directory

Understanding dental terminology will speed documentation and keep communication clear. Here are some common terms for dental appliances.

Bridges. These are permanent and connect several teeth together for support. They are not removable.

Partials. Unlike bridges, partials are removable and often involve metal work to anchor them in the mouth. They are expensive to create and replace. Inmates may have a less-expensive temporary partial, sometimes called a flipper. Temporary partials solve the issue of missing teeth without extensive fitting. Temporary partials have much less metal and crafting. Documenting that a partial is a temporary can be very helpful should the item be lost or destroyed during incarceration.

Dentures. Solid castings of the full upper or lower set of teeth are called dentures.

Orthodontic Wires. Inmates may arrive at the facility with orthodontic wires. Standard braces are found in the middle of the teeth and are used to straighten teeth. Arch bars are found below the gum line and are placed temporarily for bone healing after facial trauma. Normally, arch bars are removed after 6 – 8 weeks, but since this usually involves an office visit and expense, many inmates do not return for removal. Arch bars can remain in the mouth. It is not required that they be removed during incarceration.

By focusing on oral assessment and developing an understanding of common and emergent dental conditions, you can solve the mystery of inmate dental conditions.

Exertional Rhabdomyolysis

The majority of our inmate patients are still fairly young. Many of the youthful inmate population spend available time in sports and bodybuilding activities. Some jails and prisons also have hazing or initiation activities created by the inmates that can include extreme exercise such as squats or push-ups. These individuals are prone to contracting exertional rhabdomyolysis (rhabdo). Correctional nurses need to be alert to the potential and respond effectively to stave off a disastrous outcome.

What Causes Rhabdo?

Rhabdo is the breakdown of muscle tissue causing an outpouring of intercellular contents including myoglobin, potassium, and creatine kinase (CK). These three elements cause the life-threatening effects of the condition. Non-traumatic rhabdo can be caused by severe over-exercise, major drug ingestion, or as a result of statin use. Many corrections-related incidents of rhabdo appear in the literature including 110 knee-bends performed as a part of an inmate hazing event, narcotic overdose, and intravenous drug use.

Silent Symptoms

Rhabdo can start innocuously and may be overlooked as delayed onset muscle soreness (DONS) from over-exertion. However, if the overly sore muscles are accompanied by brown (Coca-Cola) urine or urine irregularities such as nocturia or anuria, beware. Further assessment is warranted.

Nursing Actions

A good history and assessment is necessary, including any unusual activities over the last 48 hours and a medication review. Many of our patient population are now on statins, which can complicate exertional rhabdo. If rhabdo is suspected, labs for CK,

Chapter 8: Unusual Medical Conditions

potassium, and myoglobin should be drawn while monitoring urine output and cardiac rhythm. Under medical direction, fluids should be administered to assist the body to flush out the muscle breakdown byproducts. If not caught early enough, renal dialysis and/or cardiac interventions may be necessary.

Patient and Officer Education

One of the best nursing interventions for rhabdomyolysis is patient and officer education. Inmate bodybuilders should be aware that brown urine is a bad sign that should lead to a medical visit request. Officers should understand the adverse effects of hazing activities that might be a part of a particular inmate culture. Our aggressive and macho patient population can fall prey to competitive weightlifting challenges that go beyond rational sense, requiring intervention. Prevention or early treatment of rhabdo can avoid renal failure and life-threatening arrhythmias.

With awareness, education and vigilance, correctional nurses can reduce the chances of the life-threatening results of rhabdomyolysis.

Pepper Spray

> *A call has just come in from cellblock D. They are enroute with an inmate for evaluation after being subdued with several applications of pepper spray following an aggressive incident. Two officers also sustained minor injuries during the take-down. What should the nurse prepare to do in the pepper spray evaluation?*

Pepper spray is a popular option to subdue violent or psychotic inmates when other de-escalation methods fail. It is preferred over options of lethal force in most correctional settings. A spray of concentrated capsaicin oil incapacitates most individuals due to the noxious odor and burning eyes and skin. Concentrations of the pepper oil can range from 5 – 15% depending on the product used. Potential health impact is directly correlated to the strength of concentration. If possible, obtain information about the standard products used in your facility to assist with your post-spray assessment.

The effects of pepper spray are related to skin and eye irritation, as well as neurogenic inflammation. When pepper spray comes in contact with eyes, nose and mucous membrane, it causes involuntary eye closure and a sensation of shortness of breath. These conditions provide greater chance of apprehension and incapacitation. Officers should use the minimum amount necessary to contain the situation. However, sometimes a great deal of spray is necessary and your patient may arrive having been immersed in oil.

Take Action

Use a well-ventilated exam room to assist in eliminating respiratory effects of pepper spray. Focus on these areas when performing your evaluation and determining follow-up treatment or observation.

Respiratory. There is some indication that pepper spray is particularly hazardous to those with asthma or a current respiratory infection. Check the medical record (if available) for past history and complete a thorough respiratory evaluation. Capsaicin oil causes wheezing, dry cough, shortness of breath and gagging.

Cardiac. As some have reported acute hypertension initiated by extreme pepper spray use, a vital sign check and cardiac history should also be undertaken. Symptoms usually clear in the first hour after the incident.

Skin Irritation. Skin irritation can be intense and include burning, tingling, redness, and occasional blistering. Remove any remaining vestige of irritant by having the patient wash exposed skin with soap and water. Change any soaked clothing. Irritation should clear in 30 – 60 minutes. Cool water or an ice pack can help to relieve a burning sensation.

Eye Irritation. Redness, swelling, extreme pain, tearing, and conjunctival inflammation are experienced with direct contact of the oil on eye surfaces. Eye exposure should be treated as with any other chemical eye contact – flush with water (or normal saline) for at least 15 minutes. Your medical unit should have an eye station for this purpose. Corneal abrasion can also occur, especially if contact lenses are in place. If corneal abrasion is possible, slit lamp evaluation may be necessary.

Caution Warranted

Although the majority of your patients will recover from pepper spray incidents quickly and without need of treatment, several in-custody deaths have been attributed to the chemical. A focused nursing assessment will reveal any issues of concern. Cardiac or respiratory involvement may indicate a brief stay in your infirmary for closer observation before discharge to general population.

Prison Tattoos

Tattoos have been a part of prison culture for some time. Prison tattoos are most often obtained to identify allegiance to a particular gang. Tattoos (called Tats or Ink) can also identify skills, specialties, or convictions. Tattooing is usually forbidden in the prison system, making it a daring task as well as a potentially dangerous one.

Chapter 8: Unusual Medical Conditions

Dangers of Prison Tattooing

The major danger of prison tattooing (aside from bad art work!) is blood-borne pathogen (BBP) transmission. Typical methods for tattooing inside include use of common ball-point pen ink and crude make-shift needles. Sterilization is not performed between uses. Although most inmates fear HIV transmission, the most likely BBP is Hepatitis B. The Hepatitis B virus is extremely contagious. Hepatitis C and resulting liver damage can also be transmitted through the prison tattooing process. Other complications from prison tattooing are allergic reactions to the pigment, aggravation of existing skin diseases, or keloid scarring. You may see these conditions during a sick call visit.

Education Opportunity

If tattooing is an issue in your setting, consider adding disease transmission information about prison tattooing during the intake process. Let incoming inmates know of the dangers of submitting to the tattooing process behind bars. Other education opportunities may come during sick call or cell-side rounds. Add tattoo information to regular infection control education and information materials.

Nursing Care Dilemma

An ethical dilemma can ensue if you are asked to assess a tattoo for age. Correctional nurses have been asked to determine if a tattoo is recent (and therefore 'illegal'). This situation places the nurse in a position to be part of a punitive action. Since correctional nurses must maintain a care-giving status with inmates, alternative methods are needed for assessing and staging tattoos within the facility.

Sexual Assault

The statistics on prison rape are shocking. According to a 2013 Department of Justice study, an estimated 4.0% of state and federal prison inmates and 3.2% of jail inmates reported experiencing sexual victimization in the past year. That works out to 1 in 25 inmates. A first reaction to the information may be to assume this is inmate-on-inmate victimization, but this is only part of it. More assault is reported involving facility staff (2.4%) than inmate perpetrators (2.0%).

The Prison Rape Elimination Act (PREA) was passed by the US Congress in 2003 and legislates actions to be taken by corrections personnel to prevent and respond to sexual assaults. PREA also established a Commission to monitor the process of preventing rape in the country's jails and prisons. How can correctional nurses respond?

What is Considered Prison Rape?

Any unwanted sexual contact between inmates is considered prison rape. This can include fondling of genitalia or even instilling fear of rape. It does not necessarily have to be full penetration and does not require force to be defined as prison rape.

There is an even higher standard for staff-on-inmate sexual contact. Any sexual contact between a staff member and inmate – even if consensual – is considered prison rape and can be prosecuted. Be clear for yourself and your work-mates – there is no permissible level of sexual contact with an inmate. For example, staff members have been prosecuted and sentenced for writing sexually explicit letters to inmates.

Who is a Likely Rape Candidate?

As you might expect, studies confirm that the likely inmate sexual assault victim is young, a first-time offender, and of small build. In fact, juveniles in adult prisons have a five times higher chance of being a rape victim. If you have juveniles in your facility, keep this in mind when you are providing care. Be on the look-out for indications of them having been assaulted. Some prisons automatically take protective actions for any juveniles who have received adult sentencing. This is also true for transgender, mentally-ill, or developmentally disabled inmates. Be alert when assessing and evaluating any of these categories of inmates.

Impacting Health Care

Every one of our inmate-patients is at risk for sexual assault or rape and may seek medical treatment for it. We need to be alert to the possibility and ready to respond. Here are a few examples to consider.

- An inmate arrives in sick call with a vague complaint – she is depressed, nauseous, agitated, or exhibits other traumatic stress responses.
- While working in the segregation unit, you see a normally compliant inmate break rules toward the end of their administrative segregation stay, seemingly intent on extending his time.
- A young inmate begins covering himself with feces. After mental health evaluation, it is discovered that he uses this as a protective mechanism against repeated rapes by his cell mate.

Action You Can Take

- Be familiar with your facility's assault procedures before you are confronted with a sexual assault situation. That way you will know what mechanisms to

Chapter 8: Unusual Medical Conditions

put into action. For example, you may need to inform the shift commander. Many places have a sexual assault response team consisting of a mental health provider, law enforcement professional, and medical provider.

- Document clearly the statements made by the individual. Allow them to vent without moving into investigative mode and asking questions. Asking questions too early may cause a victim to retreat and close down.

- Arrange for a sexual assault evaluation, including a rape kit if the report is within 96 hours of the assault. A specially trained individual should perform this function as forensic evidence will be obtained. In some facilities, arrangements must be made to send the inmate-patient out to a hospital emergency room for this procedure.

- Arrange frequent mental health follow-up for post-traumatic stress responses.

Unfortunately, not all correctional officers and administrative staff consider sexual assault an important issue. You may encounter conflict in your attempts to advocate for the victim. Be reminded, and remind your corrections colleagues, that being aware of the situation and not responding is both unconstitutional (Eighth Amendment) and illegal (PREA). In addition, as nurses, we have a moral obligation to act in a rape situation. Sexual assault is not a part of the punishment. We need to respond compassionately as any prudent nurse would in a community situation.

Tasers

Joyce is working at the local county jail on Friday night when a man-down code is called for the booking area. She arrives to find an obese, disheveled male lying face-down on the floor being cuffed by one of the deputies. The booking hall looks as disheveled as the man, who is now the center of activity. Another deputy tells you that the individual had 'freaked out' during the intake process and, after attempts to de-escalate the situation, a Taser was used on him. No health screening has been completed.

Tasers, or 'stun guns', are used by many law enforcement agencies to temporarily incapacitate individuals when other, lesser de-escalations or uses of force are ineffective. Guidelines for officers and for clinicians have been published that can help correctional nurses, like Joyce, determine an assessment and plan of care for Taser activation.

Tasers, also called Electronic Control Weapons (ECW), are battery-operated hand-held units that fire two barbed electrodes up to 35 feet. These electrodes are connected to the unit by copper wires and deliver a pulse of up to 50,000 volts of electricity that temporarily disrupts electrical conduction in the body. Once jolted, the individual falls to the ground and is unable to think or move for a short period of time.

Assessing the Taser Effect

As with any medical condition, nurses need to assess the immediate and ongoing effect of the Taser shock. Disrupted electrical conduction affects all muscles causing uncontrolled contraction during the time of the impulse. Heart and brain activity should be evaluated. Assess airway, breathing, and circulation at the scene. Joyce's patient is face down with officer's weight on his back as he is cuffed. Positional asphyxia is a concern.

- Consider injuries due to the de-escalation process and any other uses of force during the event. For example, Joyce needs to evaluate for trauma caused by the fall and hear a review of the pre-Taser interventions. Get as much information as possible about the context of the event to help interpret assessment findings. For example, find out if there was extensive physical struggling with the individual prior or during the use of the Taser.

- Locate the Taser barb entry points – there will be at least two – and determine if any vital areas are affected. Special concern is needed if the barb entry is near an eye, on the face or neck, or in the breast, axilla or genital areas.

- Find out how many stuns were used in the incident and for how long. Increased risk of after-effects are found with a cumulative use of over 15 seconds.

- Discover as much about the individuals medical history as possible. Joyce did not have a medical chart in this situation, but another patient might have a chart indicating any past medical history important to the evaluation such as mental illness, heart condition, or current drug and alcohol use.

Treating the Taser Wound

Superficial skin injury and surface burns are the most frequent direct injury of Taser activation. Before making contact with your patient, be sure the Taser device is no longer active. Wear gloves and expose the two or more barbs attached to the skin. If these barbs are in any of the sensitive areas indicated above, it is strongly advised that they be removed by medical providers in an emergency room setting.

- Disconnect the darts from the Taser cartridge by bending and snapping the copper wire.

Chapter 8: Unusual Medical Conditions

- Next, grasp the frame of the dart between your thumb and index finder and pull directly up from the skin surface. This will minimize any further skin damage.

- Carefully dispose of the dart as a sharp in standard sharps container or, if needed for evidence, possibly thread the dart into the Taser cartridge and provide to the appropriate security individual.

- Inspect the wound, clean with an alcohol pad, and apply a sterile dressing. A Band-Aid is acceptable.

Monitoring At-Risk Patients

Generally speaking, healthy individuals recover quickly from a stun-gun experience without lasting effect. However, a National Institute of Justice Study found that Taser use was implicated in the death of 200 individuals. Ongoing monitoring is recommended for several high risk categories of patients:

Cardiac Disease. A weakened cardiac system may not withstand a Taser shock. Take all reports of chest pain and shortness of breath seriously. EKG monitoring may be advisable for those with a history of arrhythmias.

Pregnancy. Pregnant or potentially pregnant females need added attention. In the former, obstetric evaluation soon after the event is warranted. In the latter, pregnancy testing should be performed.

Medical/Mental Health Crisis. The electrical voltage of Taser activation can exacerbate a crisis situation. An individual in active crisis due to amphetamine drug use, asthma, or excited delirium can tip over the edge after this intervention.

The use of Tasers has decreased officer and suspect injury but is not without risk. Correctional nurses who work in facilities that employ this technology are called upon to assess and treat the physical results of deployment. Joyce had a busy Friday night but her patient pulled through the experience without incident due to her assessment and interventions.

Summary

Many new correctional nurses feel like they arrived in a strange land with a head full of straw. This patient population can present with many unfamiliar medical conditions. The correctional environment also includes some unusual emergency situations. Like the Scarecrow heading down the Yellow Brick Road, correctional nurses need to find a brain to deal with every possibility.

Chapter 9: Frequent Mental Health Issues

If you work in corrections, you need to understand the basics of mental health conditions and treatments. For one thing, so many of our patients have a mental disorder. Estimates are that nearly 25% of inmates have a serious mental illness, while over half report at least one mental condition. Secondly, even if you are providing nursing care for a medical condition, a co-occurring mental health condition can affect the nurse-patient relationship. Mental illness adds complexity to any symptom interpretation and additional potential for medication interactions. Correctional nurses administering medication need to know the reason for the medications they are providing to their patients, along with the effect and side effect profiles of an array of psychotropics. Finally, correctional nurses are regularly the only health care staff in the facility when a mental health crisis is identified by officers.

Although correctional nurses are in contact with patients having many types of mental health conditions, an understanding of three primary categories of diagnoses will greatly improve the effectiveness of nursing practice in this setting. Roseann Harmen, in the Mental Health chapter of the *Essentials of Correctional Nursing*, provides this quick guide. Psychotic Disorders: Hallucinations, Delusions, Schizophrenia, thought disorders

- Antisocial Personality Disorders
- Mood Disorders: Bipolar disorder, Depression
- Traumatic Brain Injury
- Post-Traumatic Stress Disorder

This basic list can be used as a foundation for developing nursing skill in dealing with the mentally-ill patient.

Emergencies: A Deputy Calls with an Inmate "Going Nuts"

Correctional nurses may be called to deal with an urgent mental health need such as an inmate out of control in the housing units. Consider this jail scenario.

A deputy calls to say he has an inmate who is "going nuts." He wants someone to come up and "do something" about this. The inmate is a 23 year-old white male having many prior short stays in the jail without incident. This is the first time he has been held over with a charge of reckless driving. Anna, the nurse staffing the jail for this evening shift, is unfamiliar with the patient and with the deputy.

What is going on here? How should the nurse respond to this crisis? In a situation like this, the first step is to gather information to rule out a treatable medical condition that might be causing this patient response. This nurse is preparing to contact a provider but she needs to first have all the necessary information to share with the on-call nurse practitioner. She collects her emergency bag and takes a couple of minutes to see if there is any medical record on the patient before heading to the housing unit.

Medical Conditions that Cause a Psychiatric Response

While gathering subjective and objective data for an assessment, it is a good idea to have in mind the medical conditions that could be causing this response. There are several medical or organic causes of psychiatric symptoms – the two most notable are dementia and delirium tremens. This patient's age and history do not support dementia but delirium from alcohol withdrawal is a consideration. In fact, psychiatric psychosis and alcohol withdrawal delirium are easily and frequently confused. Here is a helpful guide taken from an Academy of Family Physicians article that differentiates the three conditions.

Delirium

- Rapid onset
- Visual hallucinations, disorientation, agitation, impaired attention

Dementia

- Chronic slow onset
- Disorientation and agitation

Psychosis

- Usually a slow onset
- Usually oriented, visual hallucinations rare, auditory hallucinations more common

Another consideration when gathering assessment data is the physical condition of the patient. Patients in substance withdrawal to the point of delirium will be

Chapter 9: Frequent Mental Health Issues

physically sick while dementia or psychosis will not likely present that way. The nurse needs to have all this information available to make a good clinical judgment about actions to take.

Safety Check – Always!

No matter what psychiatric condition is being evaluated, patient and staff safety is always at the forefront. Anna needs to be continually evaluating this patient's potential for harm to self or others during the assessment process.

The SAFER Model for dealing with potentially violent patients should be part of interventions with a potentially violent patient:

- S = Stabilize the situation by lowering stimuli, including voice.

- A = Assess and acknowledge the crisis by validating the patient's feelings and not minimizing them.

- F = Facilitate the identification and activation of resources (mental health staff, officers, chaplain).

- E = Encourage the patient to use resources and take actions in his or her best interest.

- R = Recovery and referral – Leave the patient in care of a responsible professional.

Anna was able to use a calming voice tone and actions to obtain needed assessment findings. This patient was indeed ill, having insomnia, nausea, and diarrhea. He began hallucinating only recently and the initial screening in the chart indicated no past history of mental or chronic illness. Anna continually reoriented the patient to reality. While awaiting a call back from the nurse practitioner, with the assistance of security staff, she was able to relocate him from the noisy housing unit to an infirmary bed for closer observation and decreased stimulation.

A Medical Condition Rather than a Discipline Issue

Thankfully, the deputy in this case sought a medical solution to this inmate outburst rather than a disciplinary one. This may be due to a collegial and collaborative relationship among staff and management in both custody and health care disciplines. It makes a difference. By contacting medical for help, the correct treatment was provided. This inmate was, indeed, withdrawing from alcohol and in delirium tremens. Through the deputy's initiation of evaluation and the nurse's astute assessment, the patient was started on a benzodiazepine; first with a high dose to get the blood level up and then tapered to response. He successfully recovered from the delirium during a short hospital stay. He was referred to substance dependency community services on release from the jail.

Psychotic Disorders: My Patient is Hearing Voices!

Psychotic patients have lost touch with reality and have unusual thought disturbances such as hallucinations and delusions. The most common psychotic disorder is schizophrenia, but patients can manifest any variety of psychotic symptoms without having this diagnosis. The Bureau of Justice reports that 15% of those in prison and 24% of those in jail reported having thought disturbances such as hallucinations or delusions. So, correctional nurses are likely to provide nursing care to psychotic patients. Consider this scenario.

> *Melinda is conducting nursing sick call in a local jail. Her next patient submitted a slip indicating right ankle pain. She interviews the patient; asking about the initiation, duration, and quality of the pain while examining the patient's ankle. The patient explains that he hears voices at night talking about the tracking device implanted in his ankle. When it is turned on he gets a sharp pain that lasts for about 20 minutes. He knows that his movements are being tracked by the government. This patient has been in the jail for 5 days. The initial screening form only indicates that the patient is not suicidal and has no history of medical or mental health treatment.*

Auditory hallucinations are one of the most common types of psychiatric symptoms. Most often these false perceptions manifest as voices but they can also be clicks, music, or other sounds. Like this patient's presentation, psychotic disorders can include both hallucinations and delusions. A delusion involves a false personal belief that the patient continues to believe even after proof to the contrary. Here is a short list of common delusion types.

- **Control.** Belief that objects or persons have control over him. This patient has a control delusion.

- **Grandeur.** An exaggerated sense of importance or power. This delusion can be combined with religiosity. ("I am Jesus Christ.")

- **Persecution.** Belief that others intend the patient harm. This patient also expresses a persecution-type delusion.

- **Reference.** Irrational belief that all objects and actions refer to the patient. "All the articles in this magazine are talking about me in code."

Chapter 9: Frequent Mental Health Issues

- **Somatic.** Delusions based on body function. A 65 year-old woman saying "I know I am pregnant even though the Dr. says I am not."

Labeling the delusion, however, is not as important as accurately describing what the patient is hearing and experiencing.

An earlier post discussed ruling out medical conditions that might cause psychiatric symptoms – particularly delirium. Melinda plans to discuss this with the on-call physician once she has gathered all the data. She knows this patient will likely need a referral to a mental health professional. The mental health nurse practitioner sees patients two afternoons a week. She won't be in until tomorrow afternoon, though, so what should Melinda do to help this patient right now?

Subjective and Objective Findings

Melinda still needs to perform a physical assessment and document subjective and objective findings. Although it is unlikely that the patient has a tracking device implanted in his ankle, he may actually be feeling pain and may have an injury. Always fully evaluate a patient concern.

In addition, exposure to medications or drugs and medical conditions such as hepatic disease or electrolyte imbalance can cause psychotic symptoms. There is little known about this patient's history. Melinda may be able to obtain helpful background information from the patient or, if available, the patient's family.

Determine Harm to Self or Others

When a patient reports hearing voices, the underlying cause can be variable: auditory hallucinations, thoughts characterized erroneously as "voices," or an indicator of malingering. Regardless, if a patient reports hearing voices, it is important to fully evaluate how this might affect the patient's safety and the safety of those around him. Ask the patient what the voices are saying and attempt to get a full range of the content. If there is any indication that the voices instruct the patient to harm himself, perform a full suicide evaluation. If the voices instruct the patient to harm others, the patient needs to be isolated from other inmates until there is a full mental health evaluation and therapy is active.

General Tips for Working with Psychotic Patients

It can be challenging to handle a patient interaction with someone who is not in touch with reality. There are a few things that Melinda was keeping in mind when communicating with this patient.

- Avoid touching the patient without warning. Although we avoid touching anyway in corrections, touch happens during assessment and vital sign readings.

- Maintain an attitude of acceptance to encourage the patient to fully share the delusion or hallucination.

- Do not reinforce the hallucination. For example, refer to an auditory hallucination as 'the voices' rather than 'they'.

- If appropriate, as when a patient is hearing the hallucination in your presence, respond truthfully in an affirming tone. Such as "Even though the voices are real to you, I do not hear them."

- Do not argue or deny a false belief. Instead, present a 'reasonable doubt' position such as "I understand that you believe this, but I am personally having a hard time accepting it."

- Avoid laughing, whispering, or talking quietly to other staff around the patient.

- Maintain an assertive, matter-of-fact, and genuine approach.

Therapy Options

Once Melinda fully evaluated the patient, she contacted his mother who was indicated on the intake form as an emergency contact. With the patient's permission, she asked his mother about his prior medical history and discovered that the patient had, indeed, been under psychiatric care in the past and had been taking risperidone (Risperdal). The patient had left home several months ago and his mother was no longer able to encourage compliance.

Armed with this information, the on-call provider was contacted and an order was obtained for this medication. Risperidone is an atypical antipsychotic agent (also called second generation) often prescribed for schizophrenia. Other drugs in this class include Clozapine (Clozaril), Olanzapine (Zyprexa), and Quetiapine (Seraquel).

Medication is not the total answer for a psychotic condition and this patient will likely need some type of therapy such as behavioral therapy, group therapy, or individual psychotherapy. Unfortunately, many settings like Melinda's have limited resources for these mental health services.

Chapter 9: Frequent Mental Health Issues

Antisocial Personality Disorders: My Patient is Lying and Manipulative

Personality is the emotional and behavioral characteristics that make up a person. Personality traits are said to be present at birth or develop early in life. Personality influences the way we see and relate to the world. Correctional patients often have disordered personalities that have led to criminality and incarceration. Although there are many forms of personality disorders such as paranoid, narcissistic, and obsessive-compulsive, the most common forms in the correctional patient populations are antisocial personality disorders. Prisoners are ten times as likely to have an antisocial personality disorder as the general population. So, correctional nurses need to understand how to recognize and respond to these conditions. Consider this patient situation:

> *Lynn is a new nurse in a medium security state prison. One morning on treatment rounds in one of the housing units she gets distracted while George is using the nail clippers. Clippers are available for use by inmates in the presence of a nurse. When she returns her attention to George the clippers are nowhere to be found and George responds "What clippers? <u>You</u> must have left them somewhere." He smiles charmingly at Lynn as she frantically searches for the missing implement. Although afraid of losing her job for carelessness, Lynn reports the situation to the housing officer who initiates a lock down and cell search. The clippers are found in George's shoe and he is placed in administrative segregation. Later it is discovered that George owed another inmate a large gambling debt and wanted moved out of general population for protection.*

Antisocial Personality Disorders (ASPD)

Antisocial personality disorders involve characteristics of social irresponsibility, exploitation of others, and lack of guilt or shame in these behaviors. These traits make ASPD patients dangerous to the emotional and psychological well-being of nurses who care for them.

What to Look For

Here is a list of common ASPD characteristics. How many of them describe patients arriving at your sick call or medication line?

- Superficial charm
- Self-centered & self-important
- Need for stimulation & prone to boredom
- Deceptive behavior & lying

- Conning & manipulative
- Little remorse or guilt
- Shallow emotional response
- Callous with a lack of empathy
- Living off others or predatory attitude
- Poor self-control
- Promiscuous sexual behavior
- Early behavioral problems
- Lack of realistic long-term goals
- Impulsive lifestyle
- Irresponsible behavior
- Blaming others for their actions
- Short-term relationships

George demonstrated several of these characteristics in the situation with Lynn. He took advantage of her and felt no shame or guilt about it. He was superficially charming while being deceptive and lying about the situation.

A patient with antisocial personality disorder, then, is manipulative, irresponsible, deceitful, and guiltless. Nurses must be careful to protect themselves while setting clear behavioral boundaries for the nurse-patient relationship.

Protect Yourself from Manipulation

Unless you are working the mental health side, your job is not to 'treat' the antisocial behavior, but to be aware of it and protect yourself. These patients will use every interaction to their advantage. They are astute at discerning another person's vulnerabilities and they prey on people who are hurting. Staff members who are lonely, insecure, or self-involved are good candidates for the manipulation of an inmate with an antisocial personality disorder. Nursing careers have ended when nurses have been drawn into sexual relationships or nefarious activities such as smuggling contraband or diverting narcotics for these individuals. Guard yourself. Know the characteristics. Keep yourself and your teammates accountable to stop potential issues before they move to a dangerous level.

Protect yourself from manipulation by treating all inmate-patients with consistent professional behavior and demeanor. Follow all security rules of conduct.

Here are a few tips.

- Don't get personal. If an inmate comments about your hair or your figure, call them on it. If the comments continue, report them.

- Do not perform even the smallest 'extra' activity for an inmate. That cotton ball or paperclip is the first step down a slippery slope.

- Treat all inmates with equal respect and professional distance. Do not show any favoritism and do not allow any in return.

- If you think you may have already been compromised, report it immediately to your supervisor and take actions to halt the progression. This may include reassignment to another care unit to break the connection.

Control the Situation

When working with ASPD patients it is important to maintain control of the situation.

- **Keep your distance**. A somewhat detached therapeutic stance will help establish the professional nature of the interaction. This patient will not appropriately respond to empathy or compassion.

- **Keep control of the relationship.** Set clear limits about your availability, frequency of encounters, and appropriate patient behavior during medical visits.

- **Keep your cool.** Monitor your own feelings when entering into a patient encounter with an ASPD patient. Be mindful of words and actions. For example, avoid responding in kind to verbal attacks or manipulation.

Establish Behavior Accountability

All patients, but those with ASPD in particular, need to be held accountable for their behavior. While it is difficult to maintain positive regard for a patient who is deceitful or manipulative, it can be done. Here are some ways to remain therapeutic in patient encounters with ASPD patients.

- Maintain an attitude that projects that it is not the patient but the patient's behavior that is unacceptable.

- When the patient exhibits unacceptable behavior, identify it as such and redirect the patient to appropriate behavior.

- Do not attempt to convince the patient to do the right thing. Instead of saying "You should" or "You shouldn't", say "You are expected to". This establishes normative behavior and depersonalizes required actions.

Interacting with patients who have ASPD can be the most frustrating part of your correctional nursing practice. However, with mindfulness toward self-protection and behavioral boundary setting, you can feel confident that you have done your best to provide quality health care in a difficult situation.

Mood Disorders: My Patient is Not Eating or Sleeping

Carrie is passing medications for the morning pill line in a large medium security state prison. One of the inmates shuffles to the window looking tired and ill. She asks the inmate "How are you doing?" as she prepares his prescribed medication and he says he can't eat or sleep since he got here 3 weeks ago because the others on the unit are so noisy and the food is terrible. Carrie knows both those things to be true but she is concerned about how ill this patient is looking and schedules him for Mental Health Clinic later that afternoon. After completing pill line she lets the mental health nurse know that she is concerned about this patient's mental state and thinks he should be evaluated for a medical or mental health condition that might be causing his symptoms.

Being incarcerated is a downer in and of itself, but Carrie is wise to have this patient evaluated for something more. There are medical conditions that can lead to lack of appetite and insomnia that need ruled out. In addition, this patient might have a mood disorder.

Mood disorders are alterations in emotions that are expressed as depression, mania or both. They interfere with a person's life, troubling him or her with severe long-term sadness, agitation, or elation. The accompanying guilt, anger, and self-doubt leads to altered life activities and relationships. The primary mood disorders are bipolar disorder and depression.

Few nurses are surprised to find so many incarcerated patients struggling with depression. This mental health diagnosis is common in the general patient population but even more so in the inmate population with 20 – 30% reporting symptoms of major depression according to a Bureau of Justice report. Like depression, bipolar disorder is common among the inmate patient population with that same report indicating that more than half of interviewed inmates reported symptoms of mania in the last year. So, if you work behind bars, it is likely that you will frequently deal with patients showing symptoms of, or being in active treatment for, a mood disorder.

Rule Out Medical Conditions First

A constant theme in dealing with mental health disorders is to rule out a medical cause for the symptoms. One study of admissions to a VA psychiatric unit found that about 3% of admissions were incorrect diagnoses of symptoms as mental illness

Chapter 9: Frequent Mental Health Issues

that was actually caused by a medical condition. The top misdiagnosed medical condition in this study was hyperglycemia/diabetes, however many other medical conditions can cause depression-like symptoms such as hypothyroidism, liver disease, and anemia. This study also found that these misdiagnoses had incomplete medical histories. It is especially easy to jump right to a mental illness diagnosis if the patient already has a past history of psychiatric care. Correctional nurses can assist with the accurate diagnosis of a condition by obtaining a full medical history along with thorough documentation of subjective and objective assessment findings.

Rule Out Self-Harm

Another constant theme in dealing with mental health disorders is to consider the likelihood of patient self-harm. Suicide ideations should be considered when a mood disorder is being evaluated. In fact, depression is implicated in more suicides behind bars than any other mental health condition.

Is it Depression or Bipolar?

If your patient presents with depression symptoms, it could also be the down side of a bipolar disorder. With this condition, the patient has excessive mood swings between periods of high activity, racing thoughts, and poor impulse control (mania) and periods of intense feelings of loss and hopelessness (depression). It is important, then, to ask a potentially depressed patient about past seasons of manic activity, such as the following.

- Inflated self-esteem or grandiosity
- Decreased need for sleep
- More talkative than usual or pressure to keep talking
- Racing thoughts
- Attention easily drawn to unimportant or irrelevant external stimuli
- Excessive activity such as unrestrained buying sprees, gambling, or foolish investments

Anticipate Treatment Options

Effective treatment for mood disorders combines medication and therapy to reduce symptoms and develop responses to the condition that will return the patient to a normal level of function. Here is a handy guide to various mental health medications from the National Institute of Mental Health (NIMH).

Medication. Antidepressants are likely to be prescribed for depression while mood stabilizers are initiated for those with a bipolar condition.

Antidepressants. The most common anti-depressant medication categories are tricyclic (TCA's), selective serotonin reuptake inhibitors (SSRI's), and serotonin-norepinephrine reuptake inhibitors (SNRI's). Each have a specific side effect profile but here are common ones for all classes.

- *Slow start* – Most antidepressants have a slow start up for symptom relief – up to 4 weeks. Counsel patients to persevere through the side effects for depression relief. If there is no response in a month, a medication change may be warranted.

- *Dry mouth* – Make sure the patient has access to liquids.

- *Sedation* – If sedation is an issue, consider moving the medication to the last dose of the day. SSRI's and SRI's can cause insomnia. In this case, consider moving the medication to the morning dose.

- *Nausea* – Try to provide medication near meal time if this is an issue.

- *Discontinuation syndrome* – The abrupt discontinuation of most antidepressants can lead to dizziness, lethargy, headache, and nausea. Therefore, there should be adequate bridging of antidepressants at intake and patients new to these medications need instruction on the importance of therapy continuation.

Mood Stabilizers. Lithium is still the most popular mood stabilizing medication for a bipolar disorder, although others in use include atypical antipsychotics such as olanzapine (Zyprexa), aripiprazole (Abilify), and risperidone (Risperdal). Lithium toxicity is a real issue for these patients and can be difficult to manage in a jail or prison. Lithium levels should be closely monitored with at least weekly laboratory work. The medication should be held and the provider contacted for levels of 1.5 mEq/L or above. At these levels the following symptoms may be noted.

- Blurred vision
- Ringing ears
- Nausea and vomiting
- Severe diarrhea
- Mental confusion

Lithium levels of 3.5 can lead to seizures, coma, and cardiovascular collapse so monitoring lithium levels is vital for patient safety.

Chapter 9: Frequent Mental Health Issues

Therapy

Group and cognitive therapy can be helpful for patients with a mood disorder. Group therapy can provide a supportive environment to gain perspective on the condition while cognitive therapy can help a patient control the thought distortions and expectations that potentiate disordered moods.

> *The inmate Carrie was concerned about did have an elevated blood glucose and is being worked up for Type II Diabetes. He was evaluated for suicide potential and obtained a low score on the screening. A mood disorder was ruled out by the psychiatrist at his monthly clinic and he was entered into an inmate diabetes support group that was being piloted in the facility.*

Traumatic Brain Injury

Although an estimated 2% of the general population has sustained a traumatic brain injury (TBI) with continuing disability, a meta analysis of studies in the inmate population indicates a prevalence of over 60%. It is suggested that this condition may be under-reported for a variety of reasons. A study performed in the Washington State Correctional System found as much as 89% prevalence. That equates to 9 out of 10 of the inmate patients having some form of brain injury.

The long-term effects of TBI are memory problems, inability to focus, and poor impulse control. Inmates with this condition may respond in anger, aggression or verbal disrespect to cover for their deficits. This means that patients with TBI often show these behaviors.

- Acting out in anger or irritation
- Forgetting rules of prohibited conduct
- Not remembering where they should be or by when
- Forgetting that they cannot go into certain areas
- Increased behavioral infractions

TBI treatment focuses on symptom management and compensation for cognitive deficits. A careful intake history is an important first step to diagnosing TBI and managing symptoms. The CDC recommends that special attention be given to impulsive behaviors, violence potential, sexual behavior and suicide risk if the inmate is depressed.

Nurse interventions should focus on assisting patient to remember and follow direction.

- Speak slowly and clearly
- Give the patient time to register the information and respond
- Provide memory tools like writing down health instructions
- Give only a few directions at a time and keep it simple

Post-Traumatic Stress Disorder

The past life experiences of many incarcerated patients lead to post-traumatic stress disorder (PTSD). According to the National Institutes of Mental Health, PTSD develops after a terrifying event or when a person is regularly put in danger or in a deadly situation. Inmate patient histories frequently include physical or sexual abuse and many have been involved in violent crime. Incarcerated military veterans can also exhibit signs of PTSD. Incarceration can intensify the PTSD experience as some facilities have an inmate culture of intimidation, coercion, and victimization.

Survivor Response to Trauma

Individuals respond to trauma in various ways based on their own background, developmental phase and the type of trauma inflicted. Like the pain experience, a survivor's response to trauma is unique. However, there are commonalities of survivor responses. Here are three main categories of symptoms related to post-traumatic stress disorder (PTSD).

- **Re-experiencing the event**. Your patient may experience nightmares and flashbacks of a traumatic event. For example, a woman who had been sexually assaulted as a child may have difficulty sleeping as memories of the assault flood into her mind as she tries to relax.

- **Avoidance.** You patient may become anxious when confronted with objects or activities that can be associated with the trauma. For example, a stern command from an officer may trigger domestic violence memories. Severe manifestations of avoidance can lead to social isolation and even psychological dissociation.

- **Hyper-arousal**. Victims of trauma can also exhibit increased irritability and exaggerated responses to environmental danger signals. For example, the patient described above may run for the corner of the room screaming when given the command by the officer.

Emotional and Psychological Support Interventions

With these survivor responses in mind, you can provide emotional and psychological support for your patients who are dealing with PTSD. It can be

Chapter 9: Frequent Mental Health Issues

challenging to balance objectivity and empathy when dealing with victims of violence.

- **Establish rapport.** A patient can pick up a caring attitude and interest by facial expression and body language. Eye contact and listening show concern and establish rapport without getting personal with the patient.

- **Respect and patience.** As you listen to the patient, actively attend to being respectful and patient. This provides emotional support.

- **Help the patient express their feelings.** Traumatized patients will have difficulty finding words to communicate their distress and the details of their experience. Fear, sadness, or rage is hard to describe when the feelings are present. Helping victims give words to their feelings can be very therapeutic. Don't impose your own words on the experience but, rather, help your patient find their own words.

Counseling and Crisis Intervention

A traumatized patient will, most likely, need professional support beyond what you can provide in a brief nursing encounter. Seek out other possible interventions available in your setting. Mental health services, group therapy, peer-to-peer support, or outside resources may be part of support services that can be provided for patients with severe PTSD.

Seizure Disorders

Correctional nurses can easily become jaded about treating inmate seizure disorders. After all, many perks can be claimed by those diagnosed with the condition – including a coveted lower bunk and some real nifty medications. So, it would be easy to think that any inmate coming in with a history of seizures or appearing with seizure activity is merely 'faking it'. However, there is good reason to evaluate a seizure claim in our patient population.

More Inmates than General Population have Seizures

Around 1% of the US adult population will be diagnosed with a seizure disorder (1 in 100). In contrast, 4% of the US inmate population has a seizure disorder (1 in 25). That is a huge disparity and gives greater understanding to the frequency of seizure history or activity in our patient population. This patient community has several risk factors which increase the likelihood of seizure activities.

Head Trauma. The incarcerated have a background with greater violence and traumatic injury than the general population. In fact, recent studies indicate that

"25 – 87% of inmates report having experienced a head injury or traumatic brain injury (TBI) as compared to 8.5% in a general population reporting a history of TBI". Head trauma increases the potential for seizure disorders.

Drug and Alcohol Withdrawal. Drug and especially alcohol withdrawal can lead to seizures. These seizures are not chronic in nature and require a specific treatment regimen. Seizure activity in withdrawal can be intensified if the inmate already has a background of epilepsy or TBI. Alcohol withdrawal can increase inmate seizure activity, especially in jails.

Domestic, Child and Sexual Abuse. Past traumatic psychological stresses such as domestic, child or sexual abuse can produce a seizure disorder known as psychogenic seizures. These seizures have been described as a physical manifestation of a psychological disturbance and have received increased attention recently. Up to one third of patients sent for EEG-video diagnostics for seizures are diagnosed with the disorder. These seizures are of psychological rather than physical origin; however, they are not being 'faked'. Like other stress-induced conditions such as stuttering or fainting, psychogenic seizures are a physical response with only minor controllability from the individual. Psychogenic seizures do not respond well to epileptic medications, but rather to counseling and other psychotropics.

Treat all Seizures as Real

As health care professionals, correctional nurses must treat all seizures as valid until proven otherwise. If a witnessed event seems questionable, there are a few easy maneuvers to take in the post-seizure period including raising an arm over the chest and letting it drop (the non-seizing person will guard/the true seizing person will not) or using smelling salts (not effective for true seizing person). It is not recommended to do a sterna rub as this can cause unnecessary injury.

Excited Delirium

> *A medical emergency is called in the booking area of a large urban jail. The inmate has ripped off his clothing and is racing about, screaming profanities. Custody officers finally subdue him with Tasers and have him on the floor securing restraints when he stops breathing. Standard emergency treatment is provided without result. The inmate is pronounced dead on arrival to the local hospital. What just happened?*

Excited Delirium (ED) is a rare but deadly condition that can confront nurses working in corrections – particularly jails. Experts differ on the cause or even existence of the condition. However, evidence is mounting in favor of the diagnosis for a variety of unexpected deaths after situations similar to the one described above.

Chapter 9: Frequent Mental Health Issues

Causes of Excited Delirium

A prevailing theory is that ED is caused by overstimulation of the brain by dopamine. Cocaine, narcotics or extreme stress can cause an increase in dopamine release. Another biomarker under study is the release of heat shock proteins that leads to problems with body heat. The person's body temperature rises rapidly without regulation. This combination overpowers the heart and respiratory systems leading to sudden death.

What Does ED Look Like?

The challenge of excited delirium in the corrections environment is to quickly identify that there is a medical condition that needs controlled and treated; as well as the behavioral issue gaining attention. An individual in the throes of ED will seem superhumanly strong and intensely hysterical, resisting all attempts at restraint. Often they are pulling off clothing to reduce the overheating. They can also seem oblivious to pain and have little response to Tasers or pepper spray.

What's a Nurse to Do?

Correctional medical experts recommend maximum efforts to subdue the individual to allow immediate medical intervention. This would not be a time for officers to slowly escalate force tactics. Once subdued, benzodiazepines to reduce the agitation is the first treatment of choice. However, corrections nurses should focus on activities to speed transport to an acute care facility able to effectively manage the condition. Temperature regulation along with oximetry and cardiac monitoring are available in that setting.

Restraint Use

> *Crystal was called to the holding area of the large city jail where she works to evaluate an inmate that was just put into* a restraint chair *after refusing to follow the direction of the deputies and continually beating his head against the concrete wall of his cell. She arrives to find the man secured to a padded metal chair with belts around shoulders, forearms, lower legs, and torso. He has on a 'spit mask' as the officers reported that he was spitting at them while they restrained him. It was a distressing sight and she stopped for a moment to take a deep breath and organize her thoughts.*

Physical restraints are still used in the criminal justice system to manage unruly inmates; most often mentally-ill or substance-involved individuals who are not willing or able to follow instruction or control themselves in custody. The risk of self-harm or the harm to others may be valid reasons for a limited use of physical restraint, but the least restrictive options are recommended. Restraint such as this example, especially when it follows a violent take-down or the use of pepper spray, can result in death. Cases in Florida, South Carolina, and Georgia emphasize the concern over the use and misuse of physical restraint in corrections.

However, sometimes a restraint chair is necessary to keep both the inmate and staff safe for a short period of time, say, to be able to administer chemical restraint or to get a handle on a situation before moving forward. Most problems with the use of restraint chairs come from use as the solution to a problem rather than a short-term intervention in a larger treatment plan.

Restraint Risks

The use of force necessary to establish control of a violent and combative person, especially if this person is large, can result in broken bones or back injury. Death from physical restraint can result from asphyxiation, aspiration, cardiac arrest and other reasons. That is why continuous monitoring of a restrained inmate's health status is important from the beginning.

Immediate Nursing Action Needed!

Correctional nurses are called upon to evaluate the health status of inmates once they are restrained, such as the situation above. It can be extremely distressing to come upon a fully restrained person like this. However, nurses can disagree with the choice of action taken while still needing to provide necessary health care in the situation. Crystal needs to act now in the best interest of her patient. Here are the immediate actions she needs to take.

- Determine if the patient is physically decompensating. Take initial vital signs; especially respirations, heart rate and consciousness.
- Check that restraints are not so tight as to restrict normal chest expansion.
- Check that limb and shoulder restraints do not have the body in a poor alignment that could cause avoidable injury.
- Check for any body injury that may have resulted from the takedown. Get a report from the officer in charge about the pre-restraint experience to determine if there are any particular body areas that need specific attention.
- Establish that the patient is being continually monitored by custody staff while in restraint – this can be by video but should also include direct visualization every 15 minutes. Respirations and consciousness should be monitored.
- Establish that the patient is not accessible by other inmates who could harm him.
- Set up a regular schedule of nursing visits – every 2 hours, at a minimum.

Chapter 9: Frequent Mental Health Issues

Ongoing Nursing Actions

All the problems of immobility descend upon a fully restrained patient. Even after immediate injury is avoided there remains increasing risk of other perils as time goes on. Just like bed rest, restraint can lead to these conditions.

- Dehydration
- Deep venous thrombosis (DVT)
- Pulmonary embolism
- Pressure ulcers
- Urinary tract infections
- Neuropathy
- Muscle wasting
- Constipation

To help avoid the hazards of immobility, then, Crystal and the other nurses need to do the following at each 2 hour check.

- Monitor vital signs
- Release limbs one at a time and move each through a normal range of motion
- Check each limb for circulation and neurovascular status
- Offer fluids and toileting

All of these interventions will likely require officer assistance.

Intervene to Reduce Time in Restraint – Mental Health Consult Stat!

Crystal is doing her part in monitoring the patient's health status and preventing physical injury while in restraints, but she has an opportunity to do so much more for this patient. As a patient advocate, correctional nurses can establish rapport with officer colleagues to make suggestions and encourage interventions on behalf of the patient. Even though an inmate is restrained by order of custody, suggest a mental health consult for a treatment and management plan to deal with the behaviors that initiated the need for physical restraint. Agreement is likely if suggested in a collegial manner focused on the needs of both the patient and the officer (who will want to end continual observation as soon as possible).

In the case above, though, Crystal was unable to convince the officers of the need for a mental health evaluation. She then contacted her supervisor on call and her supervisor directed Crystal to contact the on-call mental health provider while she contacted the jail's shift commander to broker an arrangement. By the end of the shift the inmate had been started on lorazepam (Ativan ©) and was released from restraint after being moved to a seclusion cell in the protective unit. A positive outcome to a risky patient situation.

Summary

The correctional patient population has high incidence of mental illness. So, correctional nurses need foundational understanding of the assessment and treatment of these conditions. It is the rare nurse who comes to the specialty with background in all the areas of nursing practice that are part of correctional nursing. Nurses also must handle the outcomes of correctional practices in handling mentally-ill patients, such as isolation and restraint chairs.

Chapter 10: The Women and Children

Women and children are a vulnerable and often marginalized minority of the correctional patient population; especially in settings where they are housed in conjunction with adult males such as city and county jails. State and federal prison systems have facilities where the total population may be female or juvenile. If you are fortunate enough to work in such settings, there will be a primary focus on the health needs of these specialty populations. However, if you work in a mixed setting, you will need to take into consideration the unique needs of gender and youth along with the chief concerns of your majority patient population. Here is an overview of the major issues for dealing with women and minors in the criminal justice system.

Health Concerns of Women

The Netflix series "Orange is the New Black" brings to light the invisible world of women in prison. By all accounts there are more women behind bars now than in any time in US history. This phenomenon is certainly not what was intended when the movement toward gender equity gained steam in the 1970's. Although women still constitute less than 10% of the inmate population, their numbers are increasing at an estimated rate of 5% per year.

Women entering jails and prisons have unique socioeconomic backgrounds that result in health care needs. For example, most incarcerated women have substance abuse histories and many work in the sex trade. A national profile of female inmates reveals a history of many difficulties.

- Disproportionately women of color
- Most likely to have been convicted of a drug or drug-related offense
- Fragmented family histories, with other family members also involved with the criminal justice system
- Survivors of physical and/or sexual abuse as children and adults
- Multiple physical and mental health problems
- Unmarried mothers of minor children
- Limited vocational training and sporadic work histories

It is not surprising, then, that women prisoners frequent health care services. Female inmates report higher rates of arthritis, asthma, cancer, diabetes, and hypertension than male inmates. Being female also brings with it reproductive conditions such as pregnancy, menopause, and sexually transmitted infections. Reproductive cancers such as breast, ovarian, and cervical must be screened-for, diagnosed and treated.

Incarcerated women also have higher rates of mental illnesses such as depression, bipolar disorders, and post-traumatic stress. Successful health care interactions require attention to relationship-building and sensitivity to the patient's traumatic past.

Our aging criminal justice facilities were originally created for the male population and continue to operate with a focus on their primary population gender. Pregnancy and menopause, challenging in normal conditions, can be brutal in poorly ventilated housing units that overheat in summer and are freezing in winter.

Reproductive Health

Twenty-five year old Joanie found out she was pregnant during routine screening on intake to the city jail. She had been picked up during a street sweep over the New Year's holiday. A series of poor decisions and an addiction to cocaine that she couldn't shake had landed her on the street, sleeping rough, and getting by sleeping at the local shelter, doing odd jobs, and some occasional prostitution. She hadn't noticed any pregnancy symptoms but was starting to feel anxious and irritable since she had been drug-free while detained.

Joanie is not unlike many women in jails and prisons. She is young, sexually active, and not paying much attention to her reproductive health. Like Joanie, many women in prison have not had regular health care, are poorly nourished and are substance-involved. The jail she entered is following the American College of Obstetricians and Gynecologists (ACOG) guidelines for care of incarcerated women in screening all females for pregnancy at intake. This practice assures adequate attention to prenatal care and accommodation of pregnancy in medical treatment decisions while detained.

Like most women entering the criminal justice system, Joanie is of childbearing age. She is in the early stages of an unplanned pregnancy and has not been regularly practicing any contraceptive method. Incarceration is an opportunity to increase her knowledge of contraception options and organize her future choices. One study in a northeastern US jail/prison system found that female inmates were more likely

Chapter 10: The Women and Children

to initiate birth control methods if information and medication was started before release. This is an interesting finding and indicates that correctional nurses should establish practices of education about contraception while women are incarcerated. Unfortunately, this is not a widespread practice.

Joanie is also going to need counseling about her options for her newly discovered pregnancy. She has a lot to think about. If she chooses to keep the baby she is likely to have a high-risk pregnancy. Poor nutrition, lack of prior health care, and drug and alcohol abuse put many incarcerated women at risk for complications during pregnancy; as can the high prevalence of sexually transmitted infection. If she wants to terminate this pregnancy she may face roadblocks while incarcerated as many facilities do not easily accommodate this procedure.

Pregnancy and Reproductive Health

Incarcerated women tend to have complicated and high-risk pregnancies due to their past medical histories, lack of prenatal care, and drug/alcohol use. Reproductive health is jeopardized by increased sexually transmitted diseases, pelvic inflammatory disease, and poor hygiene.

Six to ten percent of female inmates arrive pregnant and labor and delivery are high-risk and unpredictable. Nurses caring for female inmates need to be able to determine signs and symptoms of miscarriage, evaluate fetal heart tones and determine if a woman is in active labor requiring transfer to a hospital. Each of these situations is discussed as they are identified in actual legal cases described in a review published in the Prison Journal (see reference list).

Miscarriage. In *Ferris v. County of Kennebec* (1999) a pregnant inmate experienced vaginal bleeding and reported this to the nurse who determined that this was not a miscarriage but menstrual blood based on the patient's pulse rate. The patient was sent back to her cell where, after several hours of extreme pain and continued bleeding, she miscarried.

Any vaginal bleeding in a pregnant woman needs investigation. Although first trimester abortions are more often related to genetic abnormalities, second trimester events are linked to maternal conditions including use of cocaine and acute infections. A second trimester miscarriage can involve significant blood loss and pain. Retained fetal parts must be surgically evacuated to avoid infection. Miscarrying women need continuous monitoring and intervention. If the mother is Rh negative, RhoGAM may need to be administered. Therefore, a miscarrying pregnant inmate requires a nursing assessment and continuing progression monitoring until a medical determination is made for transfer to an acute care facility.

Ectopic Pregnancy. A young woman in custody at a large urban jail has continuing abdominal pain over a 14-hour period. She is found unresponsive in her cell and rushed to the hospital where she is pronounced dead on arrival. Autopsy reveals a ruptured ectopic pregnancy. Was this death avoidable?

Ectopic pregnancy, where a fertilized ovum implants somewhere outside the uterus, is an emergency event every correctional nurse should consider when confronted with abdominal pain in a female inmate of reproductive age. Indeed, this condition is particularly common among women with a history of genital infections or infertility. Smoking also increases risk. Therefore, the female inmate population is at increased risk for ectopic pregnancy.

Potential causes of acute pelvic pain are

- Appendicitis
- Ectopic Pregnancy
- Endometriosis
- Ovarian Cyst or Torsion
- Pelvic Inflammatory Disease

Abdominal pain caused by ectopic pregnancy can include vaginal bleeding. If pregnancy status is unknown, obtain a urine pregnancy test while contacting the physician. Patients with this condition can become unstable quickly. If a tubal rupture takes place, the pain will intensify and signs of shock such as low blood pressure and rapid thread pulse will be evident. Intraperitoneal hemorrhage can cause referred pain to the shoulder area and a very tender abdomen.

This is a medical emergency requiring fast action and immediate transport to acute care. Initiate emergency protocols which can include establishing an intravenous access and fluid loading. Seek immediate medical evaluation for any potentially pregnant patient with unexplained abdominal pain. Ruptured ectopic pregnancies are a leading cause of maternal mortality in the first trimester resulting in 10-15% of all maternal deaths. Shock and death can follow quickly and immediate stabilization and transport to emergency treatment is necessary.

Fetal Heart Tones. In *Coleman v. Rahija* (1997), the patient was known to have prior high-risk pregnancies and was transferred to the prison infirmary when she developed extreme abdominal pain. She was observed but no vital signs, vaginal exam, or fetal heart tones were documented. The patient was sent back to her cell and was later found on the floor in extreme pain. She was then transported to the hospital where she delivered prematurely.

Chapter 10: The Women and Children

Every facility detaining females should have a fetal heart monitor and all nursing staff should be familiar with when and how to use it. If a pregnant woman accesses the health unit for any reason, fetal heart tones should also be assessed. Normal fetal heart rate is 120 – 160 bpm. This rate can slow or speed up when the baby is in distress. Record fetal heart rate in the medical record and follow trending as with other vital assessment findings.

Active Labor. In *Staten v. Lackawanna County* (2008) a 6-month pregnant inmate complained of pressure in her pelvis. She was evaluated in the jail medical unit. The nurse determined she was not in active labor yet and the patient was relocated to a camera cell. Correctional officers did not respond to information from the patient that her water had broken and that the baby was crowning. The nurse did not continue to monitor the patient once she had left the jail medical unit. The baby was born in the cell.

Active labor can be difficult to determine in this patient population. Contractions that are strong and last from 45 – 60 seconds at a frequency of 3 – 5 minutes indicate the active labor stage. This is the time most women are admitted to the hospital. However, high-risk pregnancies or women with histories of difficult or precipitous labors need to be closely monitored earlier. In all cases, if a patient indicates that she is in labor, is assessed in the medical unit and sent back to her cell to progress further, she should be actively and regularly monitored by health care staff until a determination is made to admit to the hospital. It is inappropriate to have only security staff or the patient as sole monitors of labor progression.

Nurses are the first point of contact with health care in a jail or prison. Correctional nurses must initiate action when a pregnant patient appears to be in labor. The high-risk nature of the majority of pregnant inmates requires a high level of suspicion that labor may be progressing even if the woman is not in the final weeks of pregnancy.

Menopause and Osteoporosis

> *Hazel is a diminutive 56 year-old state prisoner serving a life sentence for murder. She has been incarcerated for 18 years now and recently fell on the icy path while heading to breakfast from her housing unit early one morning. She sustained Colles' fractures of both wrists. While being treated for the fractures she was also diagnosed with advanced osteoporosis.*

Not all women in prison are dealing with pregnancy and reproductive health issues. The aging of the inmate population means that an increasing number of female inmates need assistance with menopause symptoms and protection from osteoporosis. Managing these conditions in the criminal justice system may require creativity and a bit of patient advocacy. Here are some key concerns with possible nursing interventions.

- **Nutrition.** Hazel has been eating prison food for more than a decade. Unfortunately, most prison are challenged to provide a calcium-rich diet. Hazel needs counselling on the best options in both the cafeteria and commissary menus to increase her vitamin D and calcium intake. Supplementation may be necessary.

- **Exercise.** Weight-bearing exercise may not be convenient or even available. Hazel appears to be walking to various inmate activities; and that is a good start. She could benefit from support in developing an exercise program based on the prison gym and yard schedule. An in-cell exercise routine can also be established and encouraged.

- **Dry, Fragile Skin.** Lack of estrogen dries out skin and eyes which can lead to discomfort, breakdown, and infection. Saline eye drops and therapeutic lotions may be needed and possibly provided through the health care unit or placed on the commissary list.

- **Body Temperature Fluctuations.** Many prisons are not well ventilated in summer or heated in winter. Menopausal women may need layers of clothing for increased comfort.

- **Lack of Sleep.** Sleep is a difficult commodity in many prisons and menopausal women with insomnia or hot flashes may have even more trouble obtaining rest. Correctional nurses can help patients establish good sleep hygiene habits and possibly provide natural sleeping aids such as melatonin through the commissary.

Watch Those Kids! Children in Adult Prisons and Jails

The Supreme Court decision on mandatory life sentencing for juveniles is a reminder to all of us that there are youth with special needs in our adult prison populations. In fact, you may have more youth in your inmate patient population than you think. A study done by researchers at the University of Texas, Austin found that 22 states and the District of Columbia allow children as young as 7 to be tried as adults and then imprisoned in adult facilities. In addition, depending on the size of the county jail system, youth may be detained in adult jails awaiting arraignment. Although it is difficult to determine the number of juveniles held in adult facilities for a number of reasons, this same study reported that in a single day in 2008 there were almost 7,000 children under age 18 being held in local jails and another 3,650 confined in adult state prisons. This is a shocking number to consider.

Here are some risky health concerns for imprisoned youth.

- **Asthma.** Asthma is the most common serious chronic condition for youth. The condition can be exacerbated by the stress of confinement and environmental triggers such as dust mites, molds, cockroaches and second-hand smoke.

- **Disordered Eating.** Body image issues in this age group can lead to disordered eating such as anorexia or bulimia. Be especially watchful for signs of disordered eating in the adolescents in your patient population.

- **Nutrition.** Adolescence is a time of great nutritional need for normal growth and development. Yet, correctional facilities are often short on lean proteins, dairy products and fresh fruits and vegetables. Help your patients learn to make good food choices and advocate for healthy options in the canteen and commissary.

- **Oral Piercings**. Piercings are popular in youth and can lead to bacterial infection, pain, swelling, and difficulty swallowing or speaking. Oral jewelry must be documented and removed at the time of intake. Look for indicators of oral piercings during health screenings.

- **Pregnancy Management.** A pregnant youth is at high risk for complications, even more so if they are lacking good nutrition and prior medical management. Adolescent pregnancy can be complicated by high rates of anemia, pre-eclampsia and pregnancy psychoses.

- **Suicide and Self-harm.** Juveniles are at high risk for suicide while in confinement. They are also prone to self-harm such as cutting and burning. Look for indications of suicide intent and self-harming with any health care encounter. Assist them in getting the help and counseling they need.

- **Victimization.** Youth are at greater risk for physical and sexual assault in an adult prison. As nurses we have opportunity to advocate for added protection for youth in an adult facility. By gaining rapport with your young patient, you are more likely to hear if they are at risk in a particular situation.

Physical Development Challenges Behind Bars

A 16 year-old female is escorted to the medical clinic in a large urban jail where she is being held for arraignment for a carjacking incident. The housing officer is concerned that she has been vomiting after meals and is now refusing to eat. She appears young for her age and is underweight for her 5'6" frame. What concerns would you have if this adolescent was under your care?

No matter the age, jail is not the healthiest of places to spend time, but the growth and development needs of adolescents far outstrip the resources in many correctional settings. Correctional nurses need to be especially focused on youth in their facilities to be sure they get the attention they need. What physical development concerns should be of high priority for your youthful patient population?

Power Food – Power Struggle

A typical correctional diet is not meant to meet health spa standards but cost constraints can make some menus downright unpalatable. Turns out our 16-year-old was not tolerating the balanced but bland higher-starch diet provided. In addition, the emotional distress of incarceration can trigger appetite loss for some. Dietary intake can be one of the few life processes still in a teen's control when behind bars. Refusing to eat or voluntarily vomiting food can be a response to a controlled environment.

Adolescents, however, need increased nutrition during growth years. Rapid development requires higher levels of protein and calcium along with zinc and iron. Some institutions provide additional milk to youthful offenders to accommodate protein and calcium needs. Food high in iron and zinc include red meats and fortified breakfast cereals. Are they available in your institution?

Young women, like the patient above, are more prone to iron deficiency. They are also prone to body-image issues that can affect nutrition. Our patient needs to be evaluated for an eating disorder considering her underweight appearance and post-meal vomiting.

Exercising Control

Even in the best of situations youth are not getting enough exercise, especially females. Prison can further reduce activity through limited time out of cell. Youth, particularly those confined in adult facilities or jails, may be wary of contact with other inmates. Encouraging and supporting exercise activities can improve adolescent health while reducing stress.

Sleeping Beauty

Besides good nutrition and increased activity, adolescents need quality sleep for growth and development. Sleep while incarcerated can be disrupted by security schedules, stress, fear, and uncomfortable surroundings. Help your youthful patients establish a sleep pattern that works in their housing unit. Provide sleep hygiene information and tailor it to your particular facility and housing unit routines.

Chapter 10: The Women and Children

Psychosocial Development Challenges Behind Bars

Psychosocial development is in full-swing during middle (15 – 17 years old) and late (18 – 21 years old) adolescence, when youthful offenders are likely a part of our patient population. This is a time when detention and association with the prison social system can have far-reaching effects. A longitudinal study published a few years back found that youth, once admitted into the juvenile justice system, were 37 times more likely to be arrested as an adult than similar kids who were not put into the system. Psychosocial development during the vulnerable adolescent years provides some insight into why this might happen.

Erikson's Stages of Psychosocial Development is a widely accepted model of progressive psychosocial human development. Using this model, we can see how the criminal justice system might negatively affect detained youth in middle and late adolescents.

Industry vs. Inferiority

Pride in accomplishment, developed from childhood through puberty, can have good results for individual identify development and self-esteem. This process can go awry, however, when youth are mixing in a criminal culture where deceit, manipulation, and bullying are often rewarded; while honesty, transparency, and kindness are socially unacceptable. In interactions with youthful offenders (really with all patients!) correctional nurses can role model and encourage positive identity development to help counteract this negative influence.

Identity vs. Role Confusion

Your adolescent patients are exploring adulthood and looking for an identity that aligns with their gifts and ambitions. This is a period of discovering who they are and their place in the world. How easy it is to take on a criminal identity when surrounded by adults or peers who, by word and action, are advocating for it. Uninformed custody professionals and even health care staff can encourage this identity selection through labeling and assumption. Regularly check your attitude toward your patient. Consider how your words and actions encourage or discourage a criminal role identity in interactions with your youthful patients.

Intimacy vs. Isolation

Young adults are exploring relationships that lead to long-term commitments. Youth confined for long periods with felons can end up in destructive relationships. The need for intimacy and belonging can lead to gang involvement as this insider suggests in an editorial about youth in adult prisons. Are there ways to encourage youth in your patient population toward healthier relationships? Possibly. Consider resources available in your facility. There may be outside groups such as dog training opportunities, educational sessions, or opportunity to engage in youth-specific programs.

What Can I Do?

Unfortunately, correctional nurses do not have the authority to change the juvenile justice system, although we have an obligation to work toward social justice and a better society. It would be easy to merely acknowledge this troubling information and focus on our various medical tasks – isn't that enough? Isn't that all we can do in this situation? Maybe so, but consider how a brief conversation or action can make a difference. We have moments in our care provision to talk with our patients. A passing word or expression of concern may have an impact – one that you may not ever see to fruition – but one that may change a life.

Consider these 5 C's of Positive Youth Development and take opportunity to encourage in one of these areas with every patient contact.

- Competence
- Confidence
- Connection
- Character
- Caring/Compassion

Summary

By considering the special concerns of the female and juvenile patient populations in your correctional setting, you can make a difference as a correctional nurse and avoid the legal concerns noted above. Correctional systems were designed for the adult male majority so women and children often miss the important medical and mental health care they need.

Chapter 11: Correctional Nurse Legal Concerns

Possibly more than any other nursing specialty, correctional nursing practice is lawsuit-prone. Our patient population, already in the criminal justice system, frequently seeks legal action when they feel they have not received rightful health care. Nurses working in the correctional setting have all the same accountability for delivering and documenting care as those working in traditional settings, along with some unique risks and liabilities that need attention. Correctional nurses must be acutely aware of malpractice and negligence concerns along with specific constitutional and civil rights issues related to the incarcerated patient.

Professional Liability Issues

A nurse hears a man-down code called overhead while returning from providing sick call in one of the housing units. When she arrives at the scene, she sees that the inmate is sprawled out on the cell floor and appears unconscious. The housing officer tells her that the inmate is breathing, so she runs back to the medical unit to get oxygen and emergency supplies. When she reaches the medical unit, she tells another nurse to activate emergency medical services as the patient will definitely be heading to the hospital. The sick call nurse returns to the housing unit with the emergency supplies, provides standard emergency treatment and, some minutes later, assists the emergency personnel to prepare the patient for transport. Three months later she is named in a malpractice lawsuit.

As professional health care providers, nurses are held to standards of practice related to our licensure. Malpractice is claimed when a professional acts, or fails to act, to the level of their professional education and skill. This is also referred to as "professional negligence" as negligence itself is a general term for carelessness or a deviation from actions that would be taken by a reasonable person in the same situation.

Components of a Malpractice Claim

Six elements must be present in a malpractice claim to prevail. All factors must be convincingly presented for the nurse to be deemed liable in a malpractice case.

Duty Owed to the Patient. Nurses owe a duty of care based on licensure and role at the time of the claim. A nurse-patient relationship is established by a nurse accepting an assignment involving the patient and continues until closure of that assignment. That closure can come when the patient is handed over to another qualified individual, as in the case of infirmary care, or when the patient is released to personal self-care, as at the conclusion of a sick call episode or release from the facility. That a duty is owed in a particular circumstance is fairly easy to establish. If a nurse is in the midst of a shift and working under a job description when presented with a patient, such as in our case above, the nurse owes a duty to the patient to respond as any prudent nurse would in a similar situation.

The nature of the duty is established by the circumstances of the incident. This can be less clear and in a court case often requires the testimony of expert witnesses of similar background. These expert witnesses base their testimony on practical experience in a similar setting but also on published standards. Standards for correctional nursing practice are published by the American Nurses Association and are structured around the nursing process. Expert witnesses may also rely on accreditation standards – in correctional settings, that would be the National Commission on Correctional Health Care Standards and the American Correctional Association Standards. Although voluntary, these standards lay out indicators of quality health care processes that may be in question in a legal claim. There are also some states that have specific state statutes and regulations that address minimum standards of care expected in the correctional setting.

Breach of Duty Owed. Once duty is established, a breach of that duty then needs to be clearly presented. The groundwork has already been laid by the expert witness(es). A breach of duty relates to action or inaction that does not meet the expected standard of care for the situation. Duty owed can be established through various, often written, sources such as:

- Standing policy, procedures and protocols
- Emergency procedures
- National guidelines and standards

Foreseeability. A successful malpractice case must also establish that the nurse should have reasonably been able to foresee that harm would come. No one has a crystal ball to see into the future and some random harm can come from nurse actions. Foreseeability establishes that the injury could have been considered and steps taken to keep the patient from harm. In our case example, a nurse was called to an emergency man-down in a housing unit and was the only health care staff on the scene. Patient abandonment was alleged as the nurse did not assess the patient or provide immediate care before leaving the scene. A prudent nurse, it was

Chapter 11: Correctional Nurse Legal Concerns

claimed, would have stayed with the patient, rendering care while an unlicensed staff member brought the equipment. The plaintiff's lawyer argued that the nurse should have foreseen that the patient would be harmed by her departure without any other health care provider left there to deliver care.

Causation. The case now moves to cause. Did the nurse's breach of established duty directly cause the injury? Causation of an injury can be multi-faceted, so narrowing down cause to the nurse's action or inaction in breach of duty may be challenging. In this case, the patient suffered a hypoxic stroke, but would the outcome have been different if the nurse had repositioned the patient and provided rescue breathing? That would be for the plaintiff's legal counsel to support through the use of medical experts with experience in a similar setting.

Injury. Physical injury must then be established. This, again, must be directly linked to the nurse's breach of duty. There are some rare exceptions here, but injury must be quantifiably physical rather than merely psychological in nature. In the case above, the nurse's abandonment must be established as the proximate cause of a physical injury to the patient. This patient was permanently disabled due to brain injury.

Damages. The final element of a malpractice allegation is that damages incurred. This infers the level of the injury to the plaintiff caused by the nurse but damages can also be ascribed in a broader manner. There are three main categories of damages sought:

- *Special damages (out-of-pocket)* – These are the primary damages of a malpractice case and are determined by actual economic loss such as lost wages, medical expenses, medications or therapy. These damages can only be claimed with proof such as receipts and bills.

- *General damages (non-economic)* – These are less quantifiable damages such as pain and suffering or emotional distress. Although receipts or bills would not be available to establish this type of damage, the plaintiff must have some evidence to support the request.

- *Punitive damages* – Punitive damages are intended to add a punishment to the defendant. If a clinician lapse is particularly egregious, or misconduct or tampering is discovered in the case, punitive damages may be high.

Although not part of the legal case, malpractice determinations are reportable and considered by State Licensing Boards for disciplinary action such as suspension or revocation of licensure.

> *In this particular case, settlement was reached before trial as so often is the case. The plaintiff was awarded a large but undisclosed settlement. Was the nurse guilty of malpractice? What do you think?*

Common Areas of Nursing Malpractice Claims

A study of nursing liability claims by a major nursing malpractice insurance provider grouped common allegations by the amount of paid indemnity (money paid out by the insurance company for the case) as well as frequency of the claim type. Although this data cuts across all nursing specialties, the top categories of malpractice claims have application for correctional nurses. Let's review these as they relate to the particular perils of the correctional nursing specialty.

Scope of Practice. Scope of practice claims brought the highest payouts. The study authors proposed that this was due to a perception by the public that practicing outside of a nurse's professional license is particularly grievous. Correctional nurses have high risk of practicing outside the scope of licensure. Our specialty practice has few boundaries. Correctional peers may have little understanding of what nurses can and cannot be asked to do. There may be pressure to limit the involvement of costly outside resources. Wanting to be helpful in a difficult situation, nurses may slip into poor practice outside licensure limits. All nurses must understand the limits of their licensure but correctional nurses, in particular, must also be willing to speak up when asked to perform outside the boundaries.

Patient Assessment. Claims in this category are frequent. Patient assessment is a major component of correctional nursing practice, as nurses are most likely the first to see the patient, and a timely assessment indicates need for monitoring, treatment or referral to another professional such as a provider, dentist or mental health specialist. The most frequent successful claims in this category were failure to properly or fully complete a patient assessment and failure to assess the need for medical intervention. Of note is a category of claims related to failure to consider or assess the patient's expressed complaints or symptoms. Correctional nurses can easily slip into a pattern of considering patient complaints to be malingering, manipulative or attention-seeking. Yet, all patient complaints and expressed symptoms must be objectively evaluated as a part of professional nursing practice.

Patient Monitoring. Once again, correctional nurses, as the primary health care staff in a correctional setting, are required to monitor patient conditions and alert providers if changes warrant treatment alterations. The highest percentage of closed claims in this category was related to failure to monitor and report changes in the patient's medical or emotional condition to the practitioner.

Treatment/Care. This was a broad category in the nursing malpractice data. It included not completing orders for patient treatment as well as delays in completing orders. Mentioned in the report was the need for effective communication among practitioners as many claims were the result of communication failures. Correctional nurses often work with providers who are

Chapter 11: Correctional Nurse Legal Concerns

only minimally on-site and must be contacted by phone for orders or evaluations. Broken communication systems or delays in communication are frequent in an on-call situation. In addition, staff nurses and providers may be unfamiliar with each other, leading to judgment concerns and unfamiliarity with style and perspective. If a provider or nurse is known to be hostile or uncivil, hesitation and delay in communication can result.

Medication Administration. Drug-related errors figure prominently in this evaluation of nursing malpractice claims. The most frequent cause of medication administration claims was giving the wrong dose of medication followed by using improper technique, and administering the wrong medication. Authors of this report noted, once again, the importance of communication, particularly in clarification of confusing medication orders before administration. Medication administration in the correctional setting has additional challenges that increase risk. Pill lines are often long and nurses can be pressured to complete medication administration quickly due to other security concerns. Cell-side medication delivery in high-security areas such as administrative segregation can lead to pre-pouring medication – an increased error risk.

Documentation Deficiencies. As expected, poor documentation of nursing care contributed to many malpractice claims against nurses. Incomplete documentation was a factor in many of the above categories and bears mention as a liability risk. Correctional nurses are often called upon to maintain documentation in less-than-ideal situations. If a physical charting system is in use, the single chart may be unavailable at the time and location of care delivery. Even electronic medical records require computer availability (of a sufficient number) and accessibility (located where care is delivered). Nurses delivering care in a disseminated system may not be able to chart until returning to the medical unit hours later.

There are many legal risks to working in a correctional setting, but nurses can greatly reduce the possibility of a malpractice claim by attending to the above areas of vulnerability.

Constitutional and Civil Rights Issues

In addition to malpractice claims, nurses working in corrections must also be aware of the constitutional civil rights of detained and sentenced patients that might be abridged in nursing practice situations. A body of judgments and class action cases has grown over the last four decades with escalation following the Supreme Court decision on *Estelle v. Gamble* in 1976. Texas prisoner J. W. Gamble injured his back working on a prison farm. He contended he was not given medical treatment and even punished for his inability to work. His suit was against W. J. Estelle, the then director of the Texas State Department of Corrections. The case moved through the lower courts and came before the Supreme Court where it was judged a violation of the Eighth Amendment's prohibition of 'cruel and unusual punishment' to not provide necessary health care to prisoners. This court decision established the standard of 'deliberate indifference to serious medical needs' as a breach of the Eighth Amendment of the US Constitution.

Deliberate Indifference Explained

Inmate Brown is suing the medical director and nurses at a county jail facility for not treating a leg ulcer that later developed osteomyelitis after release. He is charging deliberate indifference to his condition. While being confined to the jail for 10 days he did not mention the leg ulcer to any medical staff and left the facility before the required 14-day physical assessment. Does he have a case?

The term "deliberate indifference" seems almost an oxymoron. Can you really be deliberately indifferent to something? This created phrase, however, is in standard usage in correctional health care and needs to be understood as it relates to nursing practice. Deliberate indifference is defined as a professional knowing of, and disregarding, an inmate's serious medical need.

Components of deliberate indifference:

- There must be a serious medical need
- Staff must know about the serious need
- Staff must intentionally and deliberately fail to provide required treatment for that need
- This failure to treat must be shown to have caused the inmate unneeded pain or suffering or similar harm.

In the case above, staff was not aware of the leg ulcer while Mr. Brown was in custody and there is no indication that staff deliberately or intentionally refused to treat his condition. It is unlikely that his case would prevail.

Serious Medical Need

According to the Supreme Court decision in *Estelle v. Gamble*, a serious medical need is one that, if left untreated, has a risk of serious harm to the patient and can be one of two categories:

- Diagnosed by a physician as requiring treatment
- Is a need so obvious that even a lay person would know it needed medical attention

Chapter 11: Correctional Nurse Legal Concerns

Again, the case above does not meet either of the standards for serious medical need. Claims of this type are more common than you might think in our particular clinical specialty. Many such cases are brought by the inmate without legal counsel and are referred to as 'pro se' cases. Pro se means a plaintiff speaks on their own behalf without legal representation.

Three Basic Rights of *Estelle v. Gamble*

The precedent-setting Supreme Court case of *Estelle v. Gamble* established the basic rights of health care for incarcerated citizens. Many court cases over the ensuing 40 years have unpacked these rights and further described them. While reading these descriptions, consider how your nursing practice is affected by the basic principle underlying the right.

Access to Medical Care. The first provision of the Supreme Court ruling is the basic right to medical care access. If an inmate needs medical attention, this cannot be denied. There are many ways in which medical care can be passively denied. Barriers to care can be found in the structure and process of security services and health care delivery systems. For example, a facility may not have enough health care staff to meet the needs of the inmate population. If patients must wait weeks to be seen by a practitioner for an urgent condition, access to care is being hindered. This provision also covers specialists and inpatient treatment. If the medical care needed for a condition cannot be provided by on-site staff, adequate and timely access to specialists must be provided.

Care That Was Ordered. If medical staff determine that a treatment is needed and an order for the treatment or medication is written, it must be honored. Security staff or internal processes cannot hinder the required treatment nor can treatment be countermanded. Of course, accommodation of security concern is understood to be foundational and collaboration with custody staff is needed to deliver medical care in jails and prisons. An example of abridgment of this right would be for custody staff to require an inmate to report to work duty when bed rest was ordered for treatment of a sprained ankle. What Estelle v. Gamble imposes, then, is a legal duty on the part of the custodial authority to honor medical orders.

A Professional Judgment. The third medical right for inmates garnered by Estelle v Gamble is a right to a professional judgment. This right covers the need for appropriate health care staff to assess and determine medical care required by an inmate. The courts want to be sure that decisions about medical care are based on medical need and not on security need or convenience. For example, necessary care cannot be denied due to budgetary constraints or as a punishment. Health care staff cannot avoid a patient because he or she is a complainer or is obnoxious. Inmates, unlike free citizens, are not able to access other sources of care if they are not getting their needs met when incarcerated. The courts want to ensure that this does not adversely affect them. This right has significant implications for correctional nurses. Inmates cannot be avoided or disregarded because they are labeled as 'troublemakers' or 'manipulators'. Treatment cannot be denied because it is too expensive for the budget. This is not to eliminate efforts to be as cost-effective as possible in providing adequate care, however.

Section 1983

> *Subpoenas have been issued at your jail for an inmate claim that his continuing headaches were ignored and he was denied necessary treatment of his 'serious medical need'. Your risk manager and legal counsel will be meeting with staff members involved in the case, including nurses involved in triaging the sick call slips. They are referring to this as a Section 1983 case.*

When first hearing the term Section 1983, it might appear to be a reference to a date. However, 1983 is not a year but a section of the US Civil Rights Act of 1871. This act was created to protect those who were being harassed by the Ku Klux Klan following the Civil War. Section 1983 of this act is the means through which US citizens can bring forward a civil claim that their constitutionally-protected rights have been violated.

Section 1983 legal claims include false arrest, unreasonable searches, equal protection and excessive force. For correctional nursing practice, Section 1983 claims involve abridgment of the Eighth or Fourteenth Amendment to the Constitution as it relates to health care provision of prisoners or detainees. In *Estelle v Gamble (1976)* the Supreme Court ruled that denial of adequate medical care constituted "cruel and unusual punishment" as was protected against by the Eighth Amendment to the Constitution. Jail detainees are not yet prisoners being 'punished' and technically are not addressed in the Eighth Amendment. However, *Bell v Wolfish* (1979) established this same need of adequate health care for unconvicted detainees under the Fourteenth Amendment which protects due process for criminal conviction. In this case, the Supreme Court ruled that failure to provide medical care was a form of punishment imposed on an individual who had not been convicted of a crime. So, although unconvicted jail detainees and prison inmates have medical rights based on two different constitutional amendments, their medical care rights are essentially the same and legal claims of injustice are brought to court through Section 1983 of the Civil Rights Act.

A Section 1983 case is a civil rights case rather than a medical malpractice case and comes with a few peculiarities. Instead of looking to determine if the standard for nursing care was provided, a Section 1983 case is looking at the primary determinants of deliberate indifference to a serious medical need. Although a

Chapter 11: Correctional Nurse Legal Concerns

Section 1983 case can be tried in either a state or federal court, plaintiff lawyers with background in these cases tend to lean toward federal courts as federal judges are receptive to claims of constitutional rights violations. Section 1983 claims also have a longer shelf-life as medical malpractice claims are governed by state law and can have a shorter timeframe for filing. In addition, plaintiff attorneys like Section 1983 cases because their fees, if they prevail, must be covered by the defendant (if reasonable). This element of the law allows for the pursuit of 'smaller' claims that might not otherwise be considered.

Prison Litigation Reform Act

An inmate's wife was concerned about her husband's poor medical care while incarcerated in a state prison. She wanted to interest a legal firm in taking on the case and was wondering what information she would need to gather. A first recommendation is to take all steps necessary to remedy the situation through standard institutional channels. For example, had he already requested treatments through the normal sick call process or submitted grievances about his medical care?

The Prison Litigation Reform Act (PLRA) was passed in 1996 to require preliminary actions before a legal claim is heard by the court. This legislation was originally proposed to limit frivolous inmate lawsuits regarding their conditions of confinement and is limited to civil cases (not medical malpractice).

Key Points of PLRA

- **Exhaustion of Administrative Remedies.** An inmate must first use the internal grievance system to the full extent (including any appeals process) before taking legal action on a claim.

- **Mental or Emotional Injury.** Cannot be claimed without first showing physical injury.

- **Screening and Dismissal.** PLRA allows a case to be screened by the court and dismissed as frivolous even before the defense is required to reply.

- **Three-Strikes Clause.** Upfront filing fees are generally waived or greatly decreased for inmates due to poverty. However, after three prior lawsuits dismissed as "frivolous, malicious or failing to state a claim for relief", this waiver is exhausted. Further filings will require that the full fee be paid up front.

The number of lawsuits filed by inmates greatly increased from 1970 to 1995. More than 40,000 inmate claims clogged the legal system in 1995. The PLRA aimed to reduce frivolous and unnecessary inmate lawsuits by creating some boundaries on the types and frequency of legal claims. Lawsuits filed by inmates have been reduced to around 25,000 per year.

Confidentiality, HIPAA and the Correctional Nurse

An RN calls the hospital for discharge information on a patient transported back to the prison infirmary from the local hospital after his jaw was wired following an inmate brawl in the exercise yard. The emergency room nurse refused to provide any information stating it would be a violation of HIPAA. She instructs the prison RN to obtain any information she needs from the patient himself.

An NP is reprimanded for telling a housing officer that one of the inmates is a severe diabetic and needs his evening snack on time.

Confidentiality of patient health information has always been a concern for nursing. Valuing patient privacy is an ethical imperative, even in the correctional setting. In recent years, the Health Insurance Portability and Accountability Act (HIPAA) has moved health care information confidentiality to a legal concern for nurses. In particular, HIPAA regulations ensure that private health information is not released to any third party without the patient's permission.

Disclosure of medical information may be necessary for the health and safety of both the patient and the large patient community within a security facility. Officers may need to know about medical conditions or disabilities that require special equipment or scheduled appointments. Some medication side effects require additional attention or changes in work duty. Joint surgery may limit movements or abilities that security needs to be aware of. Fortunately, HIPAA regulations take into account the need for some information sharing within the correctional setting and have spelled this out in the 45 C.F.R. 164.512 (k) (5) (i) section of the code. If the correctional institution represents that such protected health information is necessary for any of the following.

- The provision of health care to such individuals
- The health and safety of such individuals or other inmates
- The health and safety of the officers or employees or of others at the correctional institution
- The health and safety of such individuals and officers or other persons responsible for the transporting of inmates or their transfer from one institution, facility or setting to another
- Law enforcement on the premises of the correctional institution

Chapter 11: Correctional Nurse Legal Concerns

- The administration and maintenance of the safety, security and good order of the correctional institution

According to this section of the HIPAA regulations, an emergency nurse can confidently share health information with the receiving nurse in the prison infirmary and a nurse practitioner can alert an officer to a health need of an inmate in his charge.

Ten Ways Correctional Nurses Can Land in Court

Correctional nurse experts Kathy Wild, RN, MPA, CCHP and Royanne Schissel, RN, CCHP, have decades of experience in the specialty as staff nurses, managers and legal nurse experts. They offer this advice based on the court cases they have been involved with. Remember, this is a list of what not to do!

#1 Don't listen to your patient's description of symptoms. Correctional nurses need to be good listeners. Although patients may embellish their symptoms at times, there is still truth in and among the various information bits being presented during a patient encounter. The goal is to find the important information that determines an accurate diagnosis and response. Listening also includes obtaining information from housing officers and family members. They can have important clues to what is going on. Disregard patient information at your own peril.

#2 Don't use your assessment skills when evaluating a patient complaint. Although tempting, malingering is not an appropriate nursing diagnosis. Once this thought is expressed it can set the mind of every other care provider going forward. Correctional nurses must guard against judgmentalism and, instead, gather subjective and objective data to confirm symptoms and establish causes when dealing with patient complaints.

#3 Don't call the doctor when you're not sure about something. Long-term correctional nurses can think they know more than the doctor they would be calling. Often the provider is not a corrections specialist or does not know the patient. The context of correctional nursing can allow nurses to drift into thinking they can handle almost anything without need of a physician.

#4 Don't take the time necessary to thoroughly document your encounter. Lawsuits come along years later and you won't remember the encounter without clear and thorough documentation. Document completely and thoroughly as close as you can to the patient encounter. The medical record is both a communication tool and a legal document. Be sure the record is legible, limited to the clinical facts and without commentary on what others have done. Charting should include a first-hand account of what was observed and what was performed for the patient. In addition, in our specialty, it is also necessary to document why a patient wasn't seen. For example, the patient may have been in court or released early.

#5 Not knowing what your nurse practice act says about your practice. Unlike traditional health care settings, nurses working in corrections may not have clear practice boundaries identified by policy, procedure, and a strong nursing organizational structure. All correctional nurses, no matter the position, must have a clear understanding of what can and cannot be done based on state licensure. Nurses can be requested to perform outside their licensure by uninformed corrections administrators, physicians and even other nurses. Just because you are able to perform a function or procedure doesn't mean that you are licensed to do it. Some nurses have a misguided impression that they must be permitted to do something since an employer requests it. This is not so.

#6 Treat your patient as an inmate. It is easy to slide into a punitive perspective in dealings with inmates. After all, some of them have learned that they can get what they want through manipulation and deceit. Yet, according to Earl Nightingale, our attitude toward others determines their attitude towards us. As nurses we are called to treat all patients with respect and dignity. We cannot disrespect or abuse the patients that we are responsible to treat.

#7 Don't share critical health care information with others. HIPAA release forms are not needed for every situation. We often need to share important health information with custody officers. Officers, especially housing officers, are part of the treatment team and need to be aware of significant medical conditions that may need early medical attention. Communication is important.

#8 Don't follow up on something because "It's not your job." Nurses are responsible for positive patient outcomes. Yet, in some correctional cultures, staff are willing to do specific tasks and no more. Some correctional settings still ascribe to a functional care delivery pattern where some nurses only perform sick call while others only perform medication administration activities. "It's not my job" is not an appropriate response where patient outcomes are concerned and does not absolve nurses from responsibility in a bad outcome where something could have been done to improve a patient condition.

#9 Don't follow current protocols. Protocols often guide nursing actions in the correctional setting. They are particularly important for nursing sick call and emergency responses. Written protocols should be available at all times and staff should know where protocols can be found. For example, the only copy of clinical protocols should not be locked in a supervisor's office. Skipping protocol steps is a frequent problem in legal cases. Referring to the protocols frequently will ensure that this does not happen. Relying on memory is not good practice. Another legal concern with protocols is keeping them updated with any new changes in practice. At a minimum, nursing protocols need to be reviewed and updated annually.

#10 Don't look for other employment when you are not happy with your job. Correctional nursing is not for everyone. The environment can be unfriendly and the patient population challenging. If you don't enjoy your work you can fall into practice patterns that can land you in court. Indications that you don't like your job can include calling inmates names, calling other staff members names, having a bad attitude or taking shortcuts with patient and staff safety. Some nurses are unable to overcome concerns that inmate patients are dangerous. Yet, you can't help a patient when you are afraid. If you see these indications in yourself, consider other nursing options. Maybe correctional nursing is not a good match for you.

Summary

Most nurses are aware of basic professional liability concerns. As professionals, nurses have a duty to the public to practice within license boundaries and provide appropriate care to patients. Common areas of nursing malpractice claims are also a concern in the correctional specialty with some particular risks due to the nature of the patient and the care environment. In addition to professional liability, correctional nurses must understand the constitutional and civil rights issues surrounding providing health care to incarcerated individuals. The Eighth and Fourteenth Amendments to the US Constitution have been cited as foundational to the rights of sentenced and detained inmates to receive necessary health care. Section 1983 of the Civil Rights Act allows inmates to make a civil claim when constitutional rights are considered violated. Although correctional nurses are under the same requirements as other nurses to keep patient medical information confidential, some health information may be shared with officers if they need to be aware of a health condition in order to participate in monitoring and seeking medical treatment for those in their charge. Correctional nurses can avoid being named in court cases by being mindful to obtain objective assessments, document treatments, communicate effectively and follow established protocols.

SECTION III

More than an Empty Tin Chest
Correctional Nurse Caring

"I'm presumin' that I could be a human if I only had a heart..." – *The Tin Man*

Dorothy, Toto, and the Scarecrow came across the Tin Man rusted in the woods while traveling along the Yellow Brick Road to the Emerald City. Once they discovered his oil can and gave his joints some lubrication he was able to tell them his story. Seems he had a hollow tin chest without a heart. He was sure he needed a heart to be human and joined the merry band in seeking out the Wizard of Oz to grant his wish.

Correctional nurses, like the Tin Man, can easily feel the pull to be less than human or empty-hearted when dealing with a patient population of known murders, rapists, and criminals. Yet, caring has been established as a core component of professional nursing practice and foundational to the nurse-patient relationship. This section explores how to care as a correctional nurse.

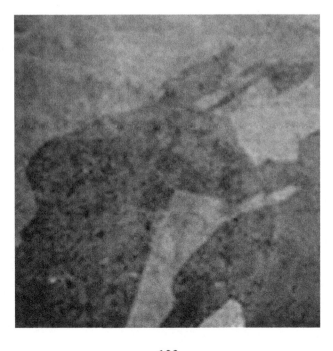

Chapter 12: Caring in the Correctional Environment

Caring for our patients is, in fact, a moral obligation to protect their health and welfare while promoting their good. We have an ethical obligation by virtue of our profession to maintain the human dignity and autonomy of our patients with whom we are in relationship. Yet, our work environment and organizational culture can militate against this duty. Many correctional nurses struggle against a tidal wave of organizational beliefs suggesting that we are caring 'too much' for our patients. Some are even derisively labeled as 'inmate lovers' or 'hug-a-thugs'.

Indeed, nurses working in jails and prisons must come to terms with how to care in the context of this work environment and patient population. We must develop a caring foundation of nursing practice that maintains the professional concept of caring while acknowledging the realities of practice in a secure setting with a stigmatized patient population deemed undesirable or untouchable.

Correctional nurses face a daily struggle to care for their patients while delivering much-needed health care in a restricted environment where they may also fear for their own personal safety. Caring for murderers, rapists, and criminals takes true grit and a more serious definition than a superficial application of a warm, positive, emotional response or empathetic word.

How can nurses truly care for and care about their inmate patient population? This is a question many in the specialty grapple with as we try to elevate the professional status of correctional nursing. Caring has been described as the essence of professional nursing practice; therefore we must establish the characteristics of this concept as it is enacted in the criminal justice system.

Weiskopf studied nurses' experience of caring for inmate patients and discovered a number of limitations in our setting. Nurses in this study described the need to negotiate boundaries between the culture of caring and the culture of custody to establish a professional relationship with custody staff in order to be effective. One surprising finding of the study was the extent to which the negative attitudes and behaviors of other nursing staff affected nurses who were attempting to provide compassionate nursing care. Many nurses working behind bars feel an obligation to care and often struggle to find ways to do this in a hostile environment. Developing a structure and process for caring may be the core defining characteristic of our specialty.

Defining Caring in Correctional Nursing

Nursing theorists have been studying the concept of caring in traditional health care settings for decades. Principles from their work can be applied to caring in the context of the criminal justice system. Here are some caring concepts from major nurse theorists and their application in the correctional setting.

Benner's Primacy of Caring

- Caring is necessary in order for a nurse to give help and for a patient to receive help.
- Connection and concern is expressed in a caring nurse-patient relationship.
- The ethic of care and responsibility guides the science of nursing.

Patricia Benner established the concept of caring as a major theme running throughout the fabric of nursing practice. It is a necessary component of the nurse-patient relationship and is seen in the actions of giving and receiving help. Correctional nurses give help in the everyday activities of sick call and emergency treatment. These, then, are not merely nursing tasks, but acts of caring. However, these actions can be delivered simply as fulfilling a job requirement. Benner further explains that caring involves connection and concern for the patient. This, then, is expressed in the desire for the patient's well-being rather than only a required task now checked off the list. This ethic of caring and responsibility to the patient guides our application of caring principles in practice.

Watson's Transpersonal Caring

- Caring involves a moral commitment to protect and enhance the patient's human dignity.
- Caring is both doing for and being with a patient who is in need.
- Caring honors the patient's dignity and vulnerability by being authentically present in the moment.

Watson's work on caring is infused with the moral implications of caring. She brings in many of the concepts of the Nurse's Code of Ethics in identifying a need to enhance and protect our patient's human dignity. This dignity is endangered every day in the correctional setting where our patients often suffer innumerable indignities as a matter of incarceration. Nurses need not add to that burden by being inconsiderate, uncivil, or disrespectful in a patient encounter. Indeed, correctional nurses are obligated to protect the human dignity of their patient

Chapter 12: Caring in the Correctional Environment

population when unnecessary compromises are being placed upon the patient population through either officer or peer action or interaction.

Leininger's Transcultural Caring

- Caring is assisting others with real or anticipated needs.
- To care is to assist, support, or enable another individual or group.
- Care must be provided in the context of the patient's culture.

Like Benner and Watson, Leininger sees caring as a necessary part of professional nursing practice that is enacted when nurses assist patients toward optimum health. A major concept for Leininger, though, is the patient's cultural perspective. Understanding a patient's cultural perspective helps a nurse to more appropriately align actions with the patient's concerns.

Considering caring within the culture of incarceration can provide an important perspective for correctional nurses. Christensen, in an article on this subject, presents some important points that support the idea that our patient population has a unique culture that should be considered for care provision. As she describes, according to Leininger, culture is the learned, shared, and transmitted values, beliefs, norms, and lifeways of a population group. Culture is learned and transmitted to those new to the group and affects the worldview of those in the group. Culture, then, guides decision-making while establishing self-worth. Reading the above description, it can be easily imagined that patients entering the criminal justice system are assimilated into a unique culture of norms, values, and beliefs that soon affects self-worth and individual decisions.

Correctional nurses need to be culturally competent to deliver effective care in the criminal justice system. This involves learning about the incarcerated culture and the affect it has on the nurse-patient relationship. Consider these cultural components that may affect patient action and decision-making.

- Inmates often participate in gangs (male) and family groups (female) that impose behavioral norms that might affect health care activities.
- There may be initiation rituals imposed on new inmates that may cause physical or psychological harm.
- Victimization can be common among inmates or by officers toward inmates.
- Inmates may believe that health care staff are equivalent to security staff and be unwilling to share personal information.
- Inmates may value group acceptance over personal health.

Tough Love is Caring, Too

Sometimes caring involves protecting a person from themselves and from the consequences of inappropriate behavior. Thus, correctional nurses care for inmate-patients by setting boundaries in the nurse-patient relationship that avoid patient harm.

Consider these unusual ways that a correctional nurses cares for patients.

- Not accepting a gift from a patient
- Letting a patient know that you know the rules and they should not ask you to violate them
- Being diligent with mouth checks during pill line

All of the examples above constitute an action or activity that is helpful for the patient; whether it avoids penalties, provides boundaries, or prevents self-harm. Caring seeks the best for the other in any situation.

Principles for Caring for Murderers, Rapists, and Criminals

Possibly one of the greatest challenges to caring in the corrections specialty is the need to care about and care for some unlovely, even monstrous, people. The very definition of professional nursing, however, requires us to consider their well-being and seek their best by preventing illness and injury while alleviating suffering. Are murderers, rapist, and criminals unworthy of our efforts? Many think so. The issue gets to the root of an ethical dilemma in our specialty and can provide insight into the very heart of nursing practice.

The ethical dilemma stems from a need to feel that our patients are worthy of our good intentions in providing nursing care. From that perspective, many behind bars do not merit our attention. But, is valuing the individual really the basis of our practice? Do we only provide nursing care to individuals who meet our moral standards or expectations? This is where the rubber meets the road in all of nursing, but it is a continual lived experience in correctional nursing.

Consider, though, that our nursing practice is more about who **we** are than about who our patients are. In other words, we choose to provide care that goes beyond any consideration of the personal attributes of our patient. That is, in fact, the first and possibly primary provision of the Code of Ethics for Nurses: "*The nurse practices with compassion and respect for the inherent dignity, worth, and uniqueness of every person.*"

Chapter 12: Caring in the Correctional Environment

Unlike those in other specialties, correctional nurses are regularly called upon to look beyond the personal attributes, social and economic statuses of our patients in order to deliver nursing care to murderers, rapists, and criminals. Yet, nurses in every area of practice, must be mindful of biases and inappropriate attitudes toward our patients. Who among us has not mentally judged a patient who is now struggling with a condition brought on by poor lifestyle choices, whether it is smoking, overeating, or alcohol intake? Have we not, even, professionalized these judgments by standardizing terms such as 'non-compliant', 'drug-seeking', or 'frequent flyer'?

Correctional nurses are daily confronted with the unique ethical nature of nursing care. It is the moral courage to *"practice with compassion and respect for the inherent dignity, worth, and uniqueness of every person"* that distinguishes professional nursing practice.

Back to the Basics

So, nurses need a heart, just like the Tin Man, to be at home in the correctional setting. By considering the context of our environment and the culture of our patient population, we can apply nursing caring concepts to our practice. Here are some basic ways that nurses enact caring behaviors in corrections.

- Educating patients about their health conditions and self-care principles
- Maintaining a nurse-patient relationship that is within the helpful zone of professional boundaries
- Advocating for the health care needs of a patient when necessary
- Showing compassion and respect
- Presenting a non-judgmental manner
- Listening to what the patient is saying
- Helping patients through a difficult situation

Can you add to this list? I'm sure, if you think about it, you can!

Summary

Some may contend that the only way to survive in the correctional setting is to have an empty tin chest; not letting emotion or feeling get in the way of nursing practice. Caring, to these nurses, is not a part of correctional nursing practice. Yet, caring is a core component of professional nursing and cannot be stripped from who we are as nurses. Thus, instead, nurses working in corrections must develop caring behaviors and attitudes that are appropriate for the correctional context and patient population. Like the Tin Man, correctional nurses still need a heart to practice effectively.

Chapter 13: Working with Inmates as Patients

Having a heart for correctional nursing also requires an honest look at our patient population. Compassion and respect for human dignity must be balanced with a practical understanding of the tendencies of our patient population and the prison culture we work within. Many of our inmate patients have lived their lives on the margins of society. These individuals have learned to deal with life, many times, through manipulation and deceit. Like an illusionist, they can distract and divert attention while accomplishing their goal. The challenge is to be ever alert to the potential for manipulation in the nurse-patient relationship without becoming jaded or cynical in dealing with our patient population.

Gary Cornelias, long time correctional leader and educator, provides helpful information to understand how to work with inmate patients in his helpful book "The Art of the Con: Avoiding Offender Manipulation". Here are some common tactics used by incarcerated patients to gain an advantage with correctional nursing staff.

- **Flattery.** Simple statements like "You look good today" or "You are the only nurse who knows what to do around here" flatter the nurse and create relationship.

- **Empathy/Sympathy.** The patient seeks to establish an identity that is 'just like you' by making empathetic comments about the work experience like "I know what you are going through. I used to have a very stressful job."

- **Helplessness.** Once a relationship is established, a request for help, other than appropriate health care, may result. Examples could include mailing a letter, gaining access to other resources, or bringing in information about a community program. These requests sound innocent, but are intended to have the nurse break some type of facility rule.

- **Sensitivity.** A patient can begin to show personal sensitivity to the nurse's condition. This may also be a ploy to create a wedge between the nurse and other staff members. "I can see how the other nurses are treating you. You deserve better."

- **Confidentiality.** The patient shares a secret with a nurse that may be inconsequential or even inaccurate but moves further into an intimate relationship and creates a bond. An example might be, "I overheard Officer Jones ask Nurse Smith for a date."

- **Isolation and Protection**. Rumor and innuendo could be shared that can lead to isolation, such as sharing that the other staff members are talking about the nurse. The patient might indicate they 'stood up for you' and protected the nurse. "I told them you were the best nurse ever and they shouldn't talk about you like that."

- **Touching.** If the verbal relationship moves along well, physical contact can start. An innocent-appearing brush of hands, tap on shoulder or body bump, if not immediately addressed, will progress to further and more frequent physical contact.

- **Sexual Innuendo**. If touching is not addressed immediately it gives the impression that it is 'OK' and sexual innuendo will follow. At this point, the nurse may be pressed for sexual favors.

- **Coercion and Intimidation**. Once a nurse has bent rules with or for an inmate-patient, coercion and intimidation can follow quickly. A nurse might be told to bring in contraband or break security rules. If refused, the inmate will threaten to reveal to the authorities the prior, more innocent actions taken. At this point the nurse has been 'hooked' by the con game and can feel trapped.

As can be seen from this list, a progression of action can take place over multiple interactions and lead to a nurse falling into the power and influence of an inmate-patient. If you see this happening to yourself or a fellow staff member, act immediately to break the progress. Stop before it gets worse. An inmate is not your friend; an inmate is your patient.

Don't Be a Target

Inmates have time on their hands and they can be a good judge of character. Unfortunately, some inmates are looking for staff member characteristics that indicate they can be manipulated and controlled. Are you a target for potential inmate manipulation? Consider which of these three staff character types best represents you.

Soft. The soft staff member wants to be liked and tries to please. This nurse is a follower rather than a leader and has difficulty saying 'No'. For example, a nurse who has joined the staff after working in a long-term care facility may be adept at comforting and accommodating patients. Soft staff members are easy prey for manipulation and often don't see it coming until they are already compromised.

Hard. The hard staff member is a no-nonsense person who follows the rules and regulations exactly. This individual is inflexible to a fault and holds themselves and

Chapter 13: Working with Inmates as Patients

others to a high standard of conduct. It would seem that a hard staff member would not be easy to compromise, but actually they have a weakness that can be exploited. So much of this staff member's self-image is wrapped up in following the rules that they can be blackmailed if even a small infraction is witnessed. Those inmates looking for a victim will seek to exploit this self-image flaw to their benefit.

Mellow. The mellow staff member also follows the rules without variation. However, this staff member understands when they need to be flexible and when they need to be firm within the confines of the system. Since their self-image is not attached to rule-keeping, they are less likely to respond to a threat of exposure and, instead, will report an inmate's threatening behavior.

A mellow staff member is difficult to turn and takes a good bit of time investment. Therefore, inmates are less likely to focus efforts on a mellow staff member. If you see characteristics of a soft or hard staff member in your self-evaluation, take steps immediately to change your behavior toward your patients.

Watch for These Techniques

Inmates who seek to manipulate and control staff members use some common techniques to select their victims and start a con. Be on guard for these behaviors in your inmate patients and don't be surprised when one of these techniques is used on you.

Inmates can intentionally target vulnerable staff members and watch for an opportunity to intervene to their benefit. They have time to watch staff members and their interactions with other staff and inmates. Conversations and actions can be carefully prepared for maximum effect. They will, in particular, seek to compromise staff by seeing how far they can be moved to break rules. Even the smallest of rule infractions can be leveraged to their advantage. Requests can include a minor contraband item such as a Band-Aid or an alcohol wipe. They may ask for medication for a headache when the rule is to request a sick call appointment. This is why it is so important to fully understand security rules and be able to interpret them in various health care interactions.

In particular, inmates will watch staff to determine weaknesses in how they perform their duties. For example, staff members will be observed for indications they are not satisfied with their job or have sloppy work habits. Staff who regularly arrive late to work, are easily distractible, or disgruntled are targets for inmate manipulation. Clothing and appearance also speak to a staff member's attention to detail and interest in professional behaviors.

Once a staff member is selected as a victim, a turn-out will begin. This can take place at an intentionally planned time or an opportunity may present itself based on a situation. In all cases, the turn-out takes place after successfully developing a relationship with staff through small requests, intimacies and favors such as 'protecting' the staff member.

Once compromised, the staff member is given a shopping list of contraband items desired by the inmate. If the victim refuses they are reminded of their many other rule infractions that will now be reported. Often staff are convinced this is a one-time request and they comply. However, this is the beginning of a long spiral downward into deeper and deeper compromise.

Once at this point, staff have three options. Many comply; some resign their positions or transfer; a few self-report. Self-report is always the best, though hardest, choice to make.

Protecting Yourself

Not all inmates are seeking victims to manipulate, but some are. Nurses working in jails and prisons need to know how to protect themselves from falling into common traps. Here are some tips to stay safe while caring for our patient population.

- Be professional at all times. Understand relationship boundaries and don't go beyond them. Some inmates will seek to gain a friendship relationship. Stay within the bounds of professional interaction.

- Be on alert when in the work environment. Be aware of those around you when you are talking about personal activities. Limit these interactions to private staff areas rather than in front of inmate patients.

- Become an expert at the games and techniques that are commonly used by manipulating inmates. Point them out to your team members when you see them. Protect each other from harm.

- Treat all patients in a firm, fair, and consistent manner. This allows little opportunity for misinterpretation or leveraging your behavior to ill advantage.

- Learn to say 'No' firmly and objectively. No need to be personal or emotional about the choice not to respond to a request.

- Keep everyone, especially your supervisor, apprised of concerns about particular inmate behaviors. Even if you have been compromised. Tell your supervisor immediately. Don't spiral further into error.

Chapter 13: Working with Inmates as Patients

- Document any compromising situation including your specific response. If there is not a formal mechanism for this documentation, keep your own personal file. This will be helpful should a particular situation come into question.

The challenge for correctional nurses is to remain caring in a therapeutic relationship without being drawn into a personal relationship and compromising security. The tightrope we walk is to deliver nursing care within the bounds of propriety and security. Your personal safety and the safety of other staff and inmates can be jeopardized if we don't get this right.

Chapter 14: Guarding Your Heart and Person

Having a heart in correctional nursing practice also requires guarding your heart, and person, from harm. Safety is a primary objective in the correctional setting. All staff members, whether health care, correctional, or support staff, should have personal safety and the safety of other team members in mind when performing job functions. Indeed, in a secure setting, safety must take precedence over therapy or treatment goals. Workplace violence, particularly violence from patients, is a main concern for correctional health care staff.

While many inmate patients are not violent, some are, and those working in the correctional setting should be ever vigilant for potential personal harm. Never become complacent about your safety while on duty in a correctional facility. Stay alert for signs of impending jeopardy and report any breach of facility safety protocol. The first step to personal safety is to know and follow all security procedures. Understand how to summon help when you feel in jeopardy and comply with all written safety instruction.

Physical Safety

Let's start with guarding yourself against physical injury. Use all your senses when monitoring personal safety, especially sight and hearing. Here are some tips for using your senses while on duty.

- Visually scan your work area and any areas you are traveling through during your work day.

- Be aware of inmate activity and always be in eyesight or hearing of a security officer when in areas accessible to inmates.

- Do not enter an area that cannot first be visually scanned prior to entry.

- Do not travel alone through areas that have blind spots or are unmonitored by security officers. Request an escort.

- Establish a standard transit route and timing with security staff for regular health care duties on your shift such as medication administration or segregation rounds. This way you will have the eyes and ears of an officer aware of your activities.

- Let others know when you are leaving the health unit and when you expect to return. Whenever possible, travel in groups or pairs rather than alone.
- Follow standard procedures for logging in and out of various areas of the facility.
- Sound is a helpful safety device. Voice can be used as a simple call for help or the facility may have alarm buttons or personal safety alarms that all staff wear.

Also be aware of your own 'sixth sense' about your personal safety. A situation may not 'feel right' even though there is not an objective reason for concern. If you feel in jeopardy, evaluate your concerns rather than over-ride them. Move to a safer location and make your concern known to officers or other staff at your location. Speak up whenever you feel unsafe.

Environmental Safety

Healthcare staff often provide assessment and treatment in an examination room. When alone with a patient in an examination room, be sure that there is always free access to the exit door. For example, position yourself between the patient and the door whenever possible. If a desk is used, have the desk positioned next to the door and the patient chair or examination table farther into the room. This avoids being blocked in the room by an angry or violent patient. Also, be aware of the alarm mechanism used in private rooms for gaining officer attention. Some rooms will have a wall alarm button to activate. Other settings may have an officer directly outside the room who can hear your raised voice if you need safety assistance.

Contraband

Another area of safety concern is contraband. This is a term used for any items not permitted into the facility or not permitted to be in the possession of the inmates. Contraband items can be used to harm others, such as a metal fork brought in with a lunch, or may be a commodity that can be sold in the prison black market, such as medications like quetiapine (Seroquel). Cell phones and drugs are particularly desirable contraband items.

Keep medications and sharps locked away from inmate access and do not be drawn in to providing your patients with any objects other than those that are necessary for care provision. Be familiar with the particular list of contraband items for the facility in which you work.

Key control is also a concern in correctional health care as many areas of activity and types of equipment and medication must be secured from inmate access. When you have responsibility for keys, be sure that they remain with you at all times. Keys

Chapter 14: Guarding Your Heart and Person

left in drawers or on counters for even short periods may result in unauthorized access to sharps and medication that can lead to personal jeopardy. Never allow inmate workers into locked areas without a staff escort.

Guard Personal Information

Personal information, in the wrong hands, can also be a safety concern. Be aware of those in the area when sharing personal information. Although talking about your life and family is a part of building rapport with your workmates, limit these types of conversations to staff-only areas such as break rooms and staff offices.

By being alert to your surroundings and careful about the personal information you share in public areas, you can contribute to your own and other staff safety. Attention to contraband and key control also helps to decrease injury risk.

Guard Your Heart by Maintaining Professional Boundaries

Professional boundaries separate therapeutic behavior in a health care relationship from other behaviors which may be well-intentioned but are not therapeutic or part of professional practice. Professional boundaries provide a defining line that protects both the patient and the care provider. They are especially important in the correctional setting as boundary violations can lead to personal and professional jeopardy. Health care staff have lost their jobs, their licenses, and even their freedom, in some cases being criminally sentenced, for violating professional boundaries with inmates.

Stay in the Zone

The National Council of State Boards of Nursing provides a helpful graphical representation of a continuum of relationship with boundaries for practice. Correctional staff must find ways to remain within the bounds of the Zone of Helpfulness in order to remain safe and provide appropriate care. Out-of-bounds relationships could include over-involvement or under-involvement.

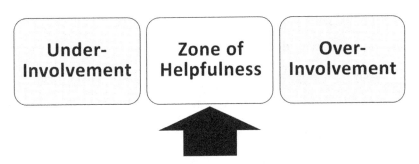

In every health care relationship, there is a power differential between the care provider's authority and the patient's vulnerability. This differential is accentuated when the patient is also an inmate with limited freedom or rights. For example, in a traditional health care situation, a patient could request a different care provider or change practices if there was discomfort or dissatisfaction. Inmates are limited to the assigned care provider's treatment.

Since health care provision is inherently personal in nature, it can be easy to drift into an intimate relationship with a patient. To guard against this drift, always maintain a relationship based on preventing illness, alleviating suffering, and protecting, promoting, and restoring the health of the patient.

Avoiding Over-Involvement

Over-involvement in a patient relationship moves toward a personal relationship that goes beyond the therapeutic role. Establishing a personal relationship with a patient is inappropriate, at best. It can be dangerous and illegal as well. Here are specific examples of professional boundary violation.

- Having a friendship relationship with a patient such as seeing them outside of a health care appointment or exchanging written communications
- Accepting or giving gifts to a patient, including providing contraband items such as cell phones or drugs
- Sexual or romantic relationships

The following list is a guide to determine if your relationship with a patient is moving toward an over-involved personal relationship. These actions indicate a boundary crossing and should be a wake-up call to re-evaluate what is going on in the patient relationship.

- Frequently thinking of the patient while away from work
- Planning your day around the care of this patient
- Sharing personal information or work concerns with the patient
- Favoring this patient's care at the expense of others
- Keeping secrets with the patient
- Selectively reporting the patient's behaviors (negative or positive)
- Changing dress style for work when working with this patient
- Acting or feeling possessive about the patient

Chapter 14: Guarding Your Heart and Person

- Swapping assignments in order to be with the patient
- Feeling responsible for the patient if progress is limited

These are the signs to look for in your own patient relationships and those of your peers. Make a pact with those you work with to call each other out if you see this behavior. Support each other in maintaining professional boundaries in your correctional practice.

Boundary crossings can happen a single time and can result from an error or lack of vigilance. A boundary violation, however, is a persistent relationship characterized by indulging in actions of a personal nature. In the correctional setting, this often involves affectionate communication – both verbal and written (love letters); sexual interaction – touch, oral sex, intercourse; or providing contraband – drugs, cell phones, alcohol.

Identifying Inappropriate Professional Behavior

We serve ourselves, our colleagues, and our patients by being alert for and responding to any indication of professional boundary crossing or violation. Five quick questions can determine if a behavior you are considering or one you observe in a colleague is within professional boundaries.

- Is the behavior consistent with your professional ethical code?
- Is the behavior consistent with your professional standards of practice?
- Is the behavior consistent with your duty to always act in the best interest of your patient?
- Does the behavior promote patient autonomy and self-determination?
- Is this a behavior you would want other people to know you have engaged in with a patient?

If the answer to any of these questions is 'No' – DON'T DO IT!!!

We all need to keep our professional boundaries in good repair and encourage our peers to do the same. Here are some recommendations for the entire health care team.

- Openly discuss the challenge of professional boundaries with your peers.
- Make a pact with your peers to 'watch their back' when it comes to observed boundary crossing. Look out for each other.
- Be particularly sensitive to stressful seasons in your personal life as this increases vulnerability to boundary violations in practice.

- Do not discuss intimate or personal issues with a patient.
- Do not keep secrets for or with patients.
- Treat all patients with dignity and respect.
- Speak, act, and dress professionally to inspire professional conduct in yourself and others.
- Be firm, fair, and consistent with all patients.
- Do not engage in behavior that can be misinterpreted as flirting, such as touching and personal compliments.

Following these guidelines will prevent boundary crossing and violation, thus protecting you and your patients from unintended consequences.

Preventing Under-Involvement

Correctional health providers can find themselves, or their peers, under-involved in patient relationships when cynicism or a jaded attitude to the inmate population takes hold. Correctional health care staff have a particular struggle to remain objective in practice. Our patient population and care environment can lead us to become skeptical and suspicious of patient complaints. New staff members soon learn that some inmates seek services for reasons other than health needs. The prison culture can value manipulation, deception, and secondary gain. Health care staff can unwittingly get caught up in a 'game' inmates are playing. Once burned in such a situation, it is easy to assume all inmates are looking for an angle when seeking health care.

Yet, many staff members have also been burned by assuming a patient is 'faking it' or being deceptive only to find that their health need was very real. What can you do to protect yourself from manipulation while also guarding against jaded cynicism?

Reasons to Be Skeptical

There are several reasons why cynicism so easily develops when dealing with our patient population.

Manipulation is a way of life. By the time many of our patients arrive in the facility, they have lived a life based on distrust, manipulation, and deception. It is how they view the world and how they have used their skills to obtain what they want.

Care may not be given if the symptoms are not severe. Some of our patients don't think they will get the attention of officers or health care staff unless they

Chapter 14: Guarding Your Heart and Person

exaggerate their symptoms. There may be a basis for their health care request but it may not be as severe as described or presented.

Health care is a way out of the facility. Other patients see health care as an opportunity to travel to the free world for hospital visits or specialty appointments. Every outside visit has the potential for contact with family and friends, or even an opportunity for escape.

Special treatment can bring status. In the stripped-down prison society, health passes for lower bunks, special shoes, or lighter work details can bring status. Special food, like evening snacks for diabetics, or desirable medications, can be used for trade or barter in the prison black market.

Special treatment can bring safety. Many inmates feel vulnerable and unsafe in general housing units. A medical or mental health diagnosis may bring a more secure housing assignment and greater safety.

Ways to Remain Objectively Caring

Those working in correctional settings must understand the very real potential of deception in the patient population while maintaining a professional perspective on the patient relationship and the need to deliver appropriate health care. Here are several ways to remain objective when dealing with inmate-patient requests.

Listen to the patient. Keep an open mind when listening to your patient. Truly hear what they are saying about their symptoms. Listen for full descriptions. Be sure to objectively document these symptom descriptions and the circumstances of their emergence. This documentation has at least two uses. First, it validates the actions you will take during this encounter. Second, it provides a history for use with ongoing encounters. If a patient is 'working the system' it can become clear over time with solid documentation of symptoms. Good communication among the health care team is important. Listening to the patient also validates concern to the patient. This may encourage accurate description of the symptom if exaggeration is an issue. Listening can help determine if safety is a concern.

Observe and document. Good observation and assessment skills are required in corrections. Document all observations with a keen eye toward those that validate or invalidate the patient's stated symptoms. Accurate and thorough observations can help the health care team 'get to the bottom' of the symptoms, whether actual or fabricated.

Seek corroborating evidence. Validation of symptoms can also be obtained from others. Officers may observe patient activities in the housing unit and the exercise yard. Other team members may have corroborating evidence. This is why an integrated medical record can be so important. Be careful, however, to limit observations to objective data. Opinions and attitudes about motivations such as using terms like 'drug-seeking' or 'malingering' have no place in the medical record.

Do not make assumptions. Even a patient who has invented illness in the past may have a serious medical need in a future encounter. It is unwise to assume that a patient is contriving the current symptoms. Every patient encounter deserves an objective evaluation.

Dealing with the Angry Patient

Workplace violence is an increasing concern in all care settings. Jails and prisons are full of angry people with poor impulse control. Correctional health care staff need skills in deflating potentially violent situations in clinical practice.

Preventing anger from escalating to violence is a primary tool to increase personal safety in this setting. The demeanor in a patient interaction can diffuse potential anger from developing. A positive assertive presence can help reduce anger escalation in a tense patient situation. Being neither aggressive nor servile in responding to an angry patient has been shown to assist in keeping the situation from getting out of hand. Three possible types of responses to anger are being aggressive, assertive, or servile. Aggressive and servile are on opposite ends of the spectrum and should be avoided, but it takes practice.

Aggressive responses to an angry patient can be risky. Aggressive responses are arrogant and make the patient feel insecure. Aggressive communication shows indifference to the causes of the situation, is commanding and uncompromising and shows a lack of concern for the patient.

On the other end of the continuum, servile responses to anger are over-cautious. A servile response seeks to placate the angry person by seeming to do what they want. This can include making unrealistic promises or unreasonable concessions. A staff member might respond to anger in this fashion when feeling intimidated. This type of response can encourage an angry patient to further escalate the anger.

A positive, assertive stance is more likely to de-escalate an anger situation. This response values the patient and aims to reduce fear. An assertive response provides guidance to the patient about the situation and attempts to negotiate a workable solution. This can have a calming effect and lead to resolution.

Tips for dealing with angry patients.
- Give extra personal space, double the usual handshake distance. This is not only calming but provides a safety buffer should things get physical.

Chapter 14: Guarding Your Heart and Person

- Listening is an action that can reduce anger. Show by both body language and conversation that you are concerned about what is causing the anger.
- Respond to the concerns of the individual using a calm tone and demeanor.
- Use mutual negotiation and shared problem solving if dealing with a rational patient.
- In all cases, engage the assistance of available corrections officers if the patient is irrational, continues to be agitated or shows any signs of physical violence.

Summary

Having a heart in correctional nursing practice is important. Guarding that heart is also necessary. Health care staff working in this setting must be proficient in skills that will maintain personal safety as well as the safety of other staff members and patients. By being mindful of facility safety procedures and work environment safety concerns, you will be able to prevent personal injury. Personal safety is also preserved by maintaining boundaries in the patient relationship. Staying within the zone of helpfulness and avoiding over- and under-involvement is key. Correctional professionals must also maintain perspective when dealing with manipulative or angry patients. Preventing anger escalation can reduce harm. By being ever mindful of your own personal safety and the safety of fellow staff members, you will prevent injury to yourself and others while delivering health care in a correctional setting with heart.

SECTION IV

The Nerve
Courage to be a Correctional Nurse

"All right, I'll go in there for Dorothy. Wicked Witch or no Wicked Witch, guards or no guards, I'll tear them apart. I may not come out alive, but I'm going in there. There's only one thing I want you fellows to do…Talk me out of it!" – Cowardly Lion

We have all felt like the Cowardly Lion of the Wizard of Oz at some time in our nursing careers. Correctional nurses, in particular, are faced with situations that require courage – moral courage – to reach patient health goals. This section explores the concept of moral courage and how it can be engaged in correctional nursing practice.

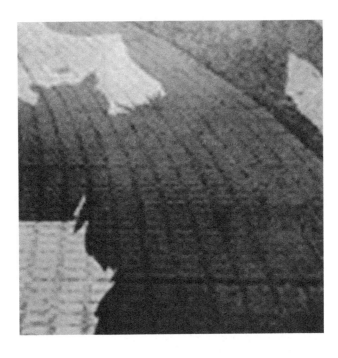

Chapter 15: Moral Courage in the Correctional Context

Correctional nurses need courage to be successful. Did you know you were courageous in accepting the challenge to work with our patient population and in our work environment? Many nurses are not that bold. They do not seek out experiences that involve security escorts, the clanging of automatic barred doors, or the need to have their personal belongings searched when entering and leaving the workplace. Yes, you are a courageous nurse!

Three Types of Courage

Courage is key to effective correctional nursing. Bill Treasurer, in his book *Courage Goes to Work: How to Build Backbones, Boost Performance, and Get Results*, describes three types of courage we need to develop. Yes, you can build your courage. It is a learnable skill like all your other nursing abilities.

TRY Courage

TRY Courage is described by Treasurer as "the courage of initiating an action— making first attempts, pursuing pioneering efforts and stepping up to the plate". TRY Courage motivates us to act when needed – even if it is hard. Have you had to advocate for the needs of one of your patients? Have you had to confront cruel or disrespectful actions of a staff member? Have you had to address inappropriate patient behavior? It takes courage.

TRUST Courage

TRUST Courage is described by Treasurer as "the courage of confidence in others— letting go of the need to control situations or outcomes, having faith in people and being open to direction and change". TRUST Courage allows us to let go of controlling the outcomes of what we do. We are responsible for right action, but can't control the outcomes of those actions. Do you have the courage to take a right action and let go of the outcome? You are a courageous nurse.

TELL Courage

TELL Courage is described by Treasurer as "the courage of voice – raising difficult issues, providing tough feedback and sharing unpopular opinions". TELL Courage is the courage to speak up when the issue is difficult or you are the only one in the situation who is disturbed. Correctional nurses are sometimes put in situations where there are no other health professionals available for consultation. Social pressure might be applied to 'go along' with the situation. Have you spoken up in a difficult situation? You are a courageous nurse.

Are you afraid to be courageous – maybe like the Lion in the forest of the Oz? The good news is that you have the capacity for gaining more courage. Fear is an invitation to courage – accept that invitation! Keep reading for some help gaining the courage you need to be a correctional nurse.

A Special Need for Moral Courage

Possibly more than any other nursing specialty, correctional nurses confront moral dilemmas in the clinical setting. Clashing worldviews of security and health care, along with the political and social implications of health care delivery to criminals, create a quagmire of ethical concerns. Many correctional nurses work in solo practices in small facilities without the benefit of a health care management structure that supports standard health care practices. Even in larger systems, ethical practices may be overruled by a security structure that is not attuned to the patient care implications of custody practices.

Moral courage is the courage to take action on a moral issue by overcoming fear of the consequences. The potential for reprisal, social isolation, and termination can lead to fear in responding to a moral issue such as patient coercion. Self-doubt can also cloud the issue. If no one else in the organization is addressing or responding to unethical or immoral practice, a nurse can question her interpretation of the situation.

Do you have what it takes to respond with courage when confronted with a similar ethical or moral issue? How can correctional nurses strengthen their moral courage?

Back to Your Roots

One way to gain moral courage is through reflection on the defining elements of our professional practice. In addressing concerns nurses can have as whistleblowers, Nurse Ethicist Vicki Lachman suggests a need to return to our professional roots. As professionals, we must be loyal to the definition of nurses as those who alleviate suffering and advocate on behalf of a patient's well-being. Therefore, as nurses, we can gain the moral courage to act in the face of unethical colleagues, patient safety violation, or fraud by reflecting on the need to report these behaviors as part of who we are as professionals.

Chapter 15: Moral Courage in the Correctional Context

Tempered with Wisdom

Moral courage in nursing practice also requires wisdom. The courageous among us can be rash in responding to what, on first review, is an unethical practice. Yet, a wise nurse considers all the facts and perspectives before sounding the alarm. A wise response is determined based on full information, while misdirected courage can lead to foolhardy actions. Wisdom tempers courage to, instead, seek the right response in any situation.

Practice Makes Perfect

Intentionally practicing moral courage can develop the skill and habit of responding even in the face of fear. Some consider courage to be equivalent to fearlessness, but that is a distortion of the concept. Courage means overcoming fear by acting in the face of adversity. By practicing the skill of overcoming small fears, a nurse can develop moral courage by progression. For example, courageously overcoming fear to respond to rude behavior from a colleague develops the moral courage muscle. Like strength training for our physical muscles, our moral courage muscle must be stressed with ever-increasing weight.

Observing Degrading Treatment

It was painful to read the account of practices in a Michigan Women's Prison where inmates were required to submit to a vaginal inspection for drug smuggling or not be permitted to receive visitors. According to the news story "Michigan's is the only prison system in the nation to routinely use such searches as a matter of policy". The International Council of Nurses (ICN) Position Statement on the nurses' role in the care of detainees and prisoners provides support for correctional nurses to respond to degrading treatment like this. The ICN Statement reads:

> *ICN believes national nurses' associations (NNA's) and individual nurses should be protected from reprisals related to advocacy for or providing care to detainees and prisoners or those who refuse to participate in torture, cruel, inhumane or **degrading treatment** (emphasis mine).*

Great strides have been made in reducing nurse involvement in practices that jeopardize the nurse-patient relationship, such as body cavity searches and collecting forensic evidence. Accrediting bodies such as NCCHC and ACA support ethical practices of informed consent and right to refuse treatment.

As patient advocates, what are the correctional nurse responsibilities to speak up and address inhumane and degrading correctional practices that are not specifically health care related? For example, what are our responsibilities for calling out degrading practices we see in an administrative segregation setting while doing nursing rounds or 'take down' procedures seen while assessing the medical condition of an inmate?

The moral distress that results from regularly observing inhumane treatment can lead to physical and mental stress-related symptoms. What can correctional nurses do in a situation where inhumane or degrading inmate treatment is witnessed? The ICN Statement suggests action is needed:

- Nurses who are aware of abuse and maltreatment take appropriate action to safeguard the rights of detainees and prisoners.

Response to Degrading Treatment

- **Speak up.** Identify to the custody officer in charge that you have concerns about a procedure that you are witnessing. Be direct, clear and calm in manner. You are expressing a professional opinion in advocating for a person in your patient population.

- **Use the chain of command.** Address your concern with your manager. Ask for guidance and support in dealing with the situation. Follow all internal policies and procedures to initiate a complaint or concern.

- **Discuss with your nurse colleagues.** If you find that an inhumane culture is pervasive in your facility, seek ways to support each other in professionally responding to individual situations from the ethical perspective of patient advocacy.

- **Ask for outside support.** Professional nursing organizations such as the American Nurses Association or your state nurse association may have additional support and advise to guide appropriate response. Make contact and request confidential advice.

As correctional nurses, we have an ethical and moral responsibility to advocate for the well-being of the patient community for which we care.

Moral Courage: Being Assertive

Speaking up in the face of a moral dilemma takes courage. No one likes conflict...well, almost no one....and nurses, it is found, would rather compromise than confront, according to at least one research study. Overcoming a natural inclination to 'go along to get along' takes conflict management skill. Like so many other nursing skills, it comes with practice. Being assertive in a moral situation is easier when assertive communication is a natural part of professional practice.

Chapter 15: Moral Courage in the Correctional Context

Knowing Me – Knowing You

Assertive communication starts with a good understanding of your own feelings about the situation and a desire to understand the feelings and perspectives of others in the group. Thoughtfully considering the situation, and your best response to it, allows an objective analysis of emotions that reduces the chance for an unhelpful aggressive or angry response.

Whenever you are distressed about a clinical situation, mentally identify your specific emotional response to become familiar with defining your feelings. Also consider the perspective of others in the situation. "Step into their shoes" and try to imagine their emotions and motivations. By evaluating all perspectives you will be prepared to assertively engage in a constructive conversation about the event.

Build-A-Response

Practicing a planned response to a situation during less significant concerns can help when the stakes are higher. One helpful model for constructing an assertive communication involves four parts.

- A non-judgmental explanation of the behavior to be changed
- An admission of the asserter's feelings
- An explanation of the tangible effect of the other person's behavior on the asserter or someone else
- Announcement of the desired behavior change solution you want, or an invitation to problem-solve.

Putting these pieces together might create a communication like this to an officer heard berating an inmate for being late to the pill line.

> *"When you call Inmate Jones a lousy pervert during pill line, I feel upset. It is demeaning and it is important to me that we are civil with each other. Could you avoid this practice?"*

By overcoming the desire to compromise and the fear of conflict, you can respond to challenging ethical situations in your correctional nursing practice. Evaluating your own feelings, seeing the perspective of others, and planning an assertive response will develop moral courage to respond when needed.

Finding the Moral Courage You Need

> *Tanya was working in a state prison in the nursing pool to make extra money for her college tuition. She was studying to be a nurse practitioner and*

thought it would be a good experience for her. Although she was learning much from her shifts there, she was also distressed by the treatment of a mentally-ill inmate in solitary confinement for striking and injuring one of the officers. Even in the short time she had been working there, she had observed significant mental deterioration. In addition, the officers were rough and rude with this inmate; she assumed due to his injuring of one of their own. Tanya was starting to lose sleep over this experience but she didn't know what to do about it.

Nurses can experience moral distress over situations they observe in the correctional setting. Moral distress is experienced when painful feelings arise over the awareness of a morally inappropriate activity but feel they cannot respond due to various obstacles. A common obstacle is that of the institution or organizational culture. This is what Tanya is experiencing. Distress can also come from the uncertainty of what action to take and what consequences might ensue. For example, could Tanya be sanctioned, rejected, ridiculed, or fired if action is taken?

Finding moral courage to overcome distress and act in the face of these potential consequences is challenging. As in an emergency situation where all-out effort is needed, nurse ethicist Vicki Lachman suggests that we should call a code. That is an acronym for a 4-step process for finding courage to act in the face of a moral dilemma.

Call a C-O-D-E when Moral Courage is Needed

	Category	Question to Ask
C	Courage to be moral	Where does my strength come from?
O	Obligations to honor	What is the right thing to do?
D	Dangers to manage	What do I need to handle my fear?
E	Expression and action	What action do I need to take to maintain my integrity?

C – Courage to be Moral

Taking a moral action requires courage. Where does the strength come from? For many nurses, the strength comes from alignment with the ethical standards of our profession. A review of the Code for Nurses can provide strength for action. Look for the particular element of the code that is in violation and ponder the

Chapter 15: Moral Courage in the Correctional Context

importance of action for your own professional integrity as well as for the good of the patient in the situation.

O – Obligations to Honor

The Code for Nurses is the ethical standard of nursing practice and establishes a nurse's patient-centered valuing that is foundational to the profession. This is the primary place to determine our obligation in a moral dilemma. However, correctional nurses work within a security framework with its own value system. It can be important to consider what values drive others involved in the situation. The Institute of Global Ethics, as described by Lachman in another source, reviewed a wide variety of ethical codes and developed a list of the 5 primary values found in all of them: honesty, respect, responsibility, fairness, and compassion. Which of these values might be motivating others in the situation? These can then be considered in working through an action plan for response.

D – Dangers to Manage

Nurses must acknowledge and manage the fear engendered in taking action in a risky situation. Successfully overcoming fear is, in fact, a definition of courage. Working through the prior steps can help in managing danger as they provide objective reasons for the action and establish the importance for proceeding. This can be powerful and should not be under-estimated.

Also suggested in the process of 'de-catastrophizing' which in involves working through the 'what ifs' of the situation. By objectifying fear, it can be demystified and balanced with the positive outcomes of action. This helps to cognitively reframe the situation and reduce negative thoughts. It also turns thoughts toward planning and action-taking rather than dwelling on fear.

E – Expression and Action

The final step in the CODE process is to take the practical action that will overcome fear and resolve the issue. Action in a situation such as Tanya's requires both assertiveness and negotiation skills. It requires an understanding of the organizational reporting structure. It requires the ability to be collaborative rather than confrontational with other disciplines.

Tanya was able to muster the moral courage to respond to her moral distress. Through her actions the inmate was re-evaluated by mental health services and a treatment plan was initiated. She continues to work at the facility and is developing collaborative relationships with her health care and custody peers. She has resolved her moral distress and feels good about the outcome.

Moral Courage: Dealing with Uncertainty

Some ethical issues are obvious and the course of action is clear. A nurse who sees that a colleague has documented administering a narcotic when the patient has not received medication requires reporting. However, correctional nurses are often faced with uncertain ethical situations that create decision stress and can lead to immobilization. A nurse who is asked to perform a blood draw for drugs may wonder if the activity will be used for a therapeutic or disciplinary outcome. Moral courage requires skill in dealing with uncertainty in an ethical situation.

Uncertainty of the Moral Situation

An uncertainty about the actual moral situation can hinder the courage to act. Consideration must be given to the actual ethical concern present. Strength for action is developed by clearly articulating the professional values that have been breached. Taking time to thoughtfully consider personal and professional valuing can help pinpoint the real issue embedded in the situation. In addition, confidentially discussing the concern with a spouse, leader, or trusted peer can lead to clarity. Sometimes putting into words the concerns of the situation give voice and vocabulary that strengthen resolve toward action.

Uncertainty of the Outcome of Action

In the C-O-D-E model for moral courage described above, the third element of this model is managing danger (D). Our uncertainty about the danger involved in acting or 'speaking up' about a potential ethical issue can be very real. Anxiety and a visceral 'fight or flight' response can ensue. How can we deal with the uncertainty of the outcome of our action?

Self-soothing. In an emotionally-charged situation, free-floating anxiety or even anger can cloud judgment and be immobilizing. Immediate stress-reduction activities can be initiated, such as taking a deep breath, slowly counting to 10, or speaking calming words to yourself like "I can do this" or "I have handled many things worse than this". These are methods of self-soothing that can help to reduce anxiety and encourage clear thinking.

Cognitive Reframing. Worry about the negative outcome of an ethical action can be reframed by actively seeking positive alternative perspectives. Although concerns about job security, peer support, or humiliation may be very real, they can be balanced by positive outcomes of taking action such as personal integrity, strength of character, and satisfaction in doing the right thing in a difficult situation.

Lachman provides a logical progression to guide action in response to fear.

Chapter 15: Moral Courage in the Correctional Context

Working through this list can help to clarify next steps in an ethically uncertain situation.

- Identify the risk you want to take
- Identify the situational fear you are experiencing
- Determine the outcome you want and what you have to do to achieve it
- Identify resources accessible to you
- Take action

Summary

Like the Cowardly Lion, correctional nurses must gain the courage to practice professionally in a difficult environment. With intentionality and practice, the muscle of moral courage can be developed to withstand the continual onslaught of challenges to the well-being of our patients and the ethical standards of our practice. Consideration of our professional ethical code and our obligations to our patients will help provide the motivation to act. Developing a support network and gaining big-picture wisdom will give us the encouragement we need to overcome fear and do the right thing.

SECTION V

Destination
Emerald City and the Wizard

"The Wizard? But nobody can see the Great Oz! Nobody's ever seen the Great Oz! Even I've never seen him!" – Guardian of the Emerald City Gates

Dorothy and her colleagues make it to the Emerald City and for a brief time think the journey is over and the Wizard will give them what they need. The Scarecrow will get a brain, the Tin Man a heart, the Lion the courage, and Dorothy will get home. But wait, after getting spruced up in the Emerald City they obtain an audience with the great and powerful Oz. Instead of giving them what they ask, Oz sends them off to obtain the Witch's broom before he will bid them their wishes. Have you ever sought an answer from a leader and, instead, got sent out with actions to accomplish rather than the solution you desired? This section has guidance for working with the Wizards in correctional nursing.

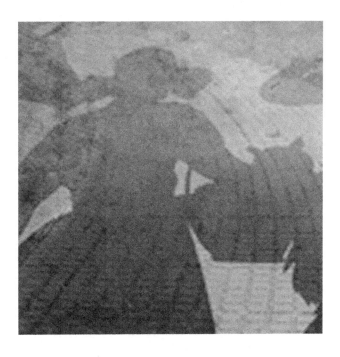

Chapter 16: Who is in Charge Here?

As discussed way back in the beginning of this story, correctional health care is delivered in an organization that has a mission of security and public safety rather than health care. To this end, the ultimate decision-makers may not be nurses or have a professional license. Correctional nurses may need to explain the goals and reasons for a desired patient outcome. In particular, the explanation must make sense within a secure environment. This might take some creativity.

The first step in reaching the goal is to find out who is in charge and how the organizational chart works. In a medium or large correctional setting, there will likely be a health services administrator or director of nursing as a front-line leader for addressing issues. In a self-operated situation, this front-line manager is going to report up through to the top leader in the facility, whether warden, sheriff, superintendent, or other title. If health care is contracted through a service provider, things get a bit more challenging. There is an organizational chart within the service company and a client relationship with the facility leadership. Facility leadership has ultimate responsibility for operations within the organization, while service provider leadership has responsibilities to facility leadership related to contractual obligations.

Next, an astute correctional nurse considers the goals of all leaders along the organizational chart when creating a defense for a change or the requested action. In particular, though, the ultimate goal of the action must contribute to the best interests of the patient. Just expect that you may need to reframe the issue in a way that is understandable to those in leadership along the chain of command.

Once the situation is framed, address it with the leader on the organizational chart directly above you. Hopefully they will be convinced that the concern needs addressed and take action. If you do not see action in progress after a reasonable timeframe, readdress the issue with your direct leader. Sometimes there are delays along the chain of command that are affecting the timeline.

What if your direct leader decides not to proceed? At this point, review the concern in your own mind and reaffirm the importance to your patient and/or patient population at the facility. You may need to consult with human resources, legal counsel, or union representation, if appropriate, to determine a next step. It is not advisable to address an issue with the next level on the organizational chart unless a patient is in imminent danger or a situation is unsafe for a patient or staff member.

Documentation is always helpful with patient concerns. Consider whether an incident report or other standardized process would allow documentation of actions you have taken in a situation. Do not, however, document a safety concern in the patient's chart unless it is directly related to the medical condition. For example, you may chart that an infirmary patient with a high risk of falls was left with the bed in low position and instructed to request assistance when needing to walk to the toilet. However, you would not chart that the bed was in poor repair and the side rails did not work. That information needs to be shared with your manager and a work requisition initiated for repair.

The Chain of Command When Things Go Wrong

Things can go very, very wrong and very quickly in a correctional setting. Correctional nurses need to know how to obtain the cooperation and support needed to do the right thing for the patient. We have an obligation to seek the best outcome for our patients in every situation. Therefore, it is essential to understand the chain of command and activate it for the patient's benefit. Often times, in a secure setting, the nurse is the only individual with the background to know that something needs done. You have an obligation to take action. If action needs to be taken quickly, initiate protection of the patient through the channels available to you in the immediate patient area. This may be the shift supervising officer or watch commander in an off-shift situation.

Imminent Patient Harm

A key component of professional nursing practice is avoiding patient harm. Nurses are charged to seek a patient's safety in delivering patient care. In a correctional setting, nurses have an additional responsibility to their general patient population. The day-to-day activities of nursing practice in the criminal justice system bring nurses into many patient experiences. For example, interactions among the inmate population and between inmates and officers may be observed while providing nursing care in housing areas or activity areas. Action must be taken in a situation where patient harm or injury may be imminent. Here are some examples of imminent patient harm that might be observed by correctional nurses.

- An inmate recently seen in nursing sick call for an enteral virus is serving in the dining hall line although a request was made for leave from that duty until cleared for return.

- An inmate is overheard being threatened by another inmate while in the medication line.

Chapter 16: Who is in Charge Here?

- A mentally-ill and asthmatic inmate is being pepper sprayed for refusing to leave his cell.

In all these situations, a correctional nurse, by virtue of knowledge and license, needs to take action to safeguard the health and safety of the patient population entrusted to his or her care.

Delays in Urgently Needed Treatment

Another area where correctional nurses may need to activate a chain of command is when urgently needed health care is being unduly delayed. Some delay may be necessary due to the security setting where paramedics may need to traverse multiple sally ports and security check points to get to a patient. Other delays may be necessary when a specialist must be contacted or extensive arrangements made for a specialized diagnostic test. The delays that require intervention, however, are those that jeopardize a patient's health and are due to inappropriate prioritizing. Here are some examples of inappropriate delays in urgently needed treatment that need leadership involvement to avoid patient harm.

- A patient being worked up for appendicitis is held in infirmary overnight until the next shift when there will be officer staff available for a transport.
- Afternoon medication line is cancelled due to an officer call-out that leaves no one available to escort the nurse to the housing unit.
- Nurse Sick Call is cancelled due to security activities such as lock downs.
- Security staff determine that an inmate experiencing an acute MI can be transported in a prison van to the local hospital instead of by EMS ambulance, because van transport will be more cost-effective.
- Nurse response to an unconscious inmate is delayed until the SWAT Team is called and assembled cell side.

Ethical Concerns

Correctional nurses must also seek higher authority when asked to perform functions that affect the integrity of the nurse-patient relationship. This can happen when officers see a task as being health care-related and do not understand the ethical responsibilities nurses have to their patients. Two basic principles of ethical care are beneficence (acting only for the benefit of the patient) and non-malfeasance (do no harm to the patient). In the course of working in a security environment, an ethical dilemma can arise when the goals of custody administration seem to conflict with these principles. Here are some common ethical situations that may require leadership involvement to avoid harm to the nurse-patient relationship.

Body Cavity Searches. Health care staff may be asked to perform searches of rectal or genital areas for contraband items such as drugs or weapons. This action would not be of benefit to the patient and has no health purpose. Professionals may have concerns that these searches done by custody might injure or harm the patient. However, there is general agreement that body cavity searches should not be performed by health care staff that have a patient-provider relationship with the inmate. Note, a body cavity search would be appropriate for a correctional nurse to perform if the patient is having symptoms indicating an overdose; possibly due to a burst drug bag inside the patient. In this case, the search and evacuation of any drugs would be of benefit to the patient in relieving symptoms.

Collecting Forensic Information. Along the same lines, requests may be made to assist with collecting forensic evidence to be used against the inmate, such as blood tests, DNA analysis or psychological evaluations. Providing such services would constitute a conflict of interest for the care providers working in the facility. Resources outside the facility medical unit should be accessed to provide these services.

Hunger Strikes. Ethical conflict can develop regarding treatment choices during hunger strikes. Most certainly, monitoring the health status of a striking inmate would be beneficent and non-malfeasant care. The dilemma begins if health care staff are asked to force feed (tube feed) the starving inmate. On one side of the issue are those who see force feeding as a way to save a patient's life. On the other side of the issue are those who see force feeding as over-riding the patient's autonomy.

Treatment Refusal/Forced Medications. A mentally competent patient has a right to refuse treatment. The nature of incarceration, however, can blur the lines of patient autonomy. Correctional nurses may be asked to administer medications to an involuntary patient. Should this happen, a determination of mental competence should be in place and a policy for forced medication followed. Custody officers cannot independently determine that medication is to be involuntarily administered. A medical or psychiatric determination must be made. Involuntary administration of a treatment or medication must be deemed necessary for the patient's good or, in some cases, for the good of the patient community; such as the need for isolation and treatment of active tuberculosis.

Inmate Discipline. Involvement in inmate discipline can also create an ethical dilemma. For the most part, health care staff should not be involved in disciplinary action or disciplinary committees determining actions in the facility in which they work. However, involvement becomes necessary when a staff member has witnessed or is the receiver of wrongful action. It is appropriate to provide factual objective testimony in order to maintain security in the facility and the safety of other inmates and staff members.

Chapter 16: Who is in Charge Here?

Witnessing Use of Force. Cell extractions and other uses of force deemed necessary by security to control inmates is clearly not an activity to involve nurse participation. Nurses may be asked to review an inmate's medical record to determine if any particular medical precaution needs to be taken into consideration such as an artificial joint or cardiac condition. Nurses should also be involved in medically evaluating an inmate following the use-of-force event. Leadership should be engaged by any correctional nurse being pressured to partake in use of force toward an inmate.

Summary

Dorothy did the right thing in going to the person in charge when she had a concern. It is important to know the chain of command and seek guidance and support when issues that seem beyond your control need attention and action. That may be the beginning, rather than the end, of a string of other actions that need to be taken. Those actions may seem to take as much courage as Dorothy needed to confront the Wicked Witch of the West and gain the broomstick. Whether imminent patient harm, delays in treatment, or ethical dilemmas, be prepared to act for the benefit of your patient.

CONCLUSION

You Have Always Had the Power!

"Come back! Come back! Don't go without me! Please come back!" – Dorothy Gale

"I can't come back, I don't know how it works! Good-bye, folks!" – The Wizard of Oz

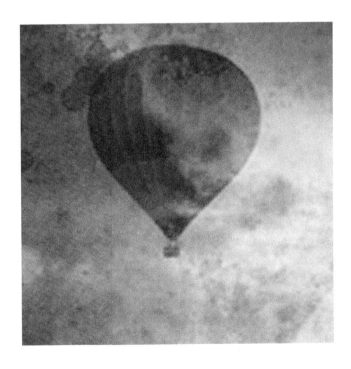

Dorothy finally made it back to the Wizard carrying the Witch's broomstick. She assumed that the Wizard would now grant her wish and send her back to Kansas. Unfortunately, the Wizard left in his hot air balloon without Dorothy. Although he turned out to be a good man, he still let Dorothy down. He was unable to take her back home with him in his balloon. Instead she was left to fend for herself. Correctional nurses can feel this way if there is poor leadership in the health care unit. Yet, like Dorothy, you can be the change you want to see in the world. Don't give up trying to do good for your patient population. You never know how your simple actions can make a difference. The Wicked Witch of the West summed this up nicely when she said of Dorothy when that bucket of water was thrown on her:

"Who would have thought a good little girl like you could destroy my beautiful wickedness?"

You may think that you are a very small cog in the great criminal justice system. You may feel that what you say or do will not matter much. Think again. People wait for a leader to step out. Be that leader that you want to see in the correctional nursing world around you. You may not be able to change everything, but you can change one little thing....and that can make all the difference. Recently two correctional nurses working in two different parts of the country shared stories of experiences with grateful inmates who noticed that they had taken the time to truly listen to their health concern and act upon it. Those nurses made a difference in the lives of their patients. You can, too!

"You have always had the power to get back to Kansas" – Glinda, the Good Witch of the South

When the Wizard left Dorothy in the Land of Oz, she wasn't sure what to do. Then Glinda, the Good Witch of the South, entered the scene. She informs Dorothy that she always had the power to get back home but that Dorothy had to learn it for herself. You, too, have the power within you to be at home in your role as a correctional nurse. In fact, you have the power within you to be a force for good in the correctional setting in which you are practicing. But, like Glinda tells Dorothy, you have to learn it for yourself. Whether through a better understanding of your work environment, patient population, language, or custody colleagues; whether through gaining knowledge, compassion, or the moral courage; whether through learning how to activate the power of the organizational hierarchy – you have the power within you to be at home in the new land of correctional nursing. You can make a difference in the lives of your patients and work colleagues. But, you need to hold on to a positive perspective on who you are and what you are doing in the criminal justice system.

Conclusion

A Little Story to Remember What You are Doing Here

Here is a short story I heard years ago that changed my life for the better. I try to remember it several times a year to help center my mental perspective. Have you heard a version of this before?

> *Two workmen were approached by a bystander on a major construction site. They were both performing the same job and were asked what they were doing. The first one said, "What does it look like I'm doing? I'm laying brick." The second one looked up from where he was crouched and off toward the sky. His response? "I'm building a cathedral."*

Two men doing the same job yet from a very different mental perspective. Which one do you think went home that night feeling like he was doing something that mattered? Which one left the worksite feeling satisfied with his lot in life?

What might you tell a visitor to your work place if they asked you what you do as a correctional nurse? Would you respond like the first workman and say, *"I pass pills and take sick call"*? Or, would you say, *"I optimize health, prevent illness and injury, and alleviate suffering."* That last answer comes from the definition of correctional nursing.

It is All About Perspective

Yes, both those workmen were doing the same thing and both had an honest response. And, both the options for describing your work as a correctional nurse would be true…but what a difference in perspective. The first perspective is of activity while the second perspective is about purpose. Thinking about purpose in our day-to-day work provides the meaning and satisfaction that makes it worth the extra effort.

Most of us become nurses to help those in need and there is not a needier patient population than inmates. So, the real effort in the correctional specialty is often to mentally balance the patient-focused purpose of our work with the ever-present struggle with a needy patient population in a challenging environment. It can really get you down.

Mind Your Mind

So, have this goal for your correctional nursing practice – Mind Your Mind. What I mean by that is to keep tabs on your attitude toward your work. This is an important goal no matter where you work, but it can be a real battle in the correctional environment. In case you haven't noticed, jails and prisons are not happy places. Most people, including many of our officer colleagues (!), don't want to be there. Hanging around with criminals all day can be a real downer. Plus, it is always necessary to be on guard for possible physical, emotional, or mental harm. No wonder you are exhausted as you walk out the sally port to the parking lot.

Take Action Right Now on This Goal

I hope you are convinced that keeping a positive mental perspective is a worthy goal for your correctional nursing practice. However, this quote says it all.

> *"A goal without a plan is just a wish" – Antoine de Saint-Exupery*

So, here are some action steps to start your "Mind Your Mind" plan.

- Establish a way to regularly remind yourself of your professional purpose. Maybe you can have it on a post-it note on your car dashboard so you can recite it on the way to work in the morning.
- On your walk from the medical unit to the facility exit, see if you can list all the ways that you improved health, prevented illness and injury, and alleviated suffering during your shift.
- On your way home, mentally close the door on all that is going on at the facility so you can truly engage with family and friends and rest during your time away from work.
- Get some form of regular mild exercise like walking or biking to help your mental perspective.
- Develop a plan to get the rest you need to be both alert and in a good mental perspective when you are at work.

Will you be building a cathedral or merely laying bricks in your correctional nursing practice? I hope you will join me in cathedral building!

Conclusion

Not the End but the Beginning!

Tell me about your journey to being at home in your correctional nursing practice. Contact me at lorry@correctionalnurse.net. Keep in touch by subscribing to my monthly newsletter at www.correctionalnurse.net/subscribe. Each issue includes highlights from my blog, podcast, news, and latest publications.

Need More on Correctional Nursing and Correctional Health Care?

Sign up for the CorrectionalNurse.Net email list for monthly news and occasional important updates: www.correctionalnurse.net/subscribe

Book List and Education Modules: www.correctionalnurse.net/lorryslist

Here are other titles available from Amazon (affiliate links)

Essentials of Correctional Nursing: www.correctionalnurse.net/essentials

The Correctional Nurse Manifesto: www.correctionalnurse.net/manifesto

The Correctional Health Care Patient Safety Handbook: www.correctionalnurse.net/handbook

About the Author

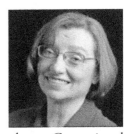

Lorry Schoenly is a nurse author and educator specializing in correctional health care. She provides consulting services to jails and prisons across the US, helping to improve professional health care practice and patient safety. Dr. Schoenly actively promotes correctional health care through social media outlets and increases the visibility of the specialty through her popular blog – CorrectionalNurse.Net. Her podcast, Correctional Nursing Today, reviews correctional health care news and interviews correctional health care leaders. She is the recipient of the National Commission on Correctional Health Care 2013 B. Jaye Anno Award of Excellence in Communication. Lorry is author of *The Correctional Health Care Patient Safety Handbook, The Correctional Nurse Manifesto*, and co-editor and chapter author of *Essentials of Correctional Nursing*, the first primary practice text for the correctional nursing specialty. She resides in the mountains of north central Pennsylvania.

References

Agency for Healthcare Research and Quality (AHRQ). (2008). *Patient safety and quality: An evidence-based handbook for nurses.* AHRQ Publication No. 08-0043. Agency for Healthcare Research and Quality, Rockville, MD. Retrieved from http://www.ahrq.gov/professionals/clinicians-providers/resources/nursing/resources/nurseshdbk/index.html

American Nurses Association (ANA). (2013.) *Correctional nursing scope and standards of practice.* Silver Springs, MD: Nursingbooks.org.

Baillergeon, J., Binswanger, I.A., Penn, J.V., Williams, B.A., & Murray, O.J. (2009). Psychiatric disorders and repeat incarceration: the revolving prison door. *American Journal of Psychiatry, 166*(1), 103-9.

Beck, A. J., & Berzofsky, M. (2013). *Sexual victimization in prisons and jails reported by inmates, 2011–12.* Bureau of Justice Statistics. Retrieved from http://www.bjs.gov/content/pub/pdf/svpjri1112.pdf

Benner, P., & Wrubel, J. (1989). *The primacy of caring: Stress and coping in health and illness.* Menlo Park, CA: Addison-Wesley.

Binswanger, I. A., Merrill, J. O., Krueger, P. M., White, M. C., Booth, R. E., & Elmore, J. G. (2010). Gender differences in chronic medical, psychiatric, and substance-dependence disorders among jail inmates. *American Journal of Public Health, 100*(3), 476-482.

Bloom, B., Owen, B., Covington, S. (2005). *Gender-responsive strategies: A summary of research, rractice, and guiding principles for women offenders.* National Institute of Corrections. Retrieved from http://static.nicic.gov/Library/020418.pdf

Carson, E. A. & Sabol, W. J. (2012). *Prisoners in 2011.* Washington, DC: Bureau of Justice Statistics. Retrieved from http://www.gutsandgore.co.uk/wp-content/uploads/2013/03/Prisoners-in-2011.pdf

Centers for Disease Control. (n.d.). *Traumatic brain injury: A guide for criminal justice professionals.* Retrieved from http://www.cdc.gov/traumaticbraininjury/pdf/Prisoner_TBI_Prof-a.pdf

Chakera, A., Cowan, N. & Winearls, C. (2008). STIR(ing) appearance of rhabdomyolysis. *Clinical Kidney Journal, 1*(5), 373-4. doi: 10.1093/ndtplus/sfn092

Chapman, A., & Dixon-Gordon, K. (2007). Emotional antecedents and consequences of deliberate self-harm and suicide attempts. *Suicide and Life-Threatening Behavior, 37*(5), 543-552.

Christensen, S. (2014). Enhancing nurses' ability to care within the culture of incarceration. *Journal of Transcultural Nursing, 25*(3), 223-231.

Clarke, J. E., Herbert, M. R., Rosengard, C., Rose, J. S., DaSilva, K. M., & Stein, M. D. (2006). Improving birth control service utilization by offering services prerelease vs postincarceration. *American Journal of Public Health, 96*(5), 840-845.

Committee on Health Care for Underserved Women. (2011). *Health care for pregnant and postpartum incarcerated women and adolescent females.* The American College of Obstetricians and Gynecologists. Retrieved from http://www.acog.org/Resources_And_Publications/Committee_Opinions/Committee_on_Health_Care_for_Underserved_Women/Health_Care_for_Pregnant_and_Postpartum_Incarcerated_Women_and_Adolescent_Females

Cornelius, G. (2009). *The art of the con: Avoiding offender manipulation* (2nd ed.). Alexandria, VA: American Correctional Association.

CorrectionsOne.com. (2014). *15 prison tattoos and their meanings.* Retrieved from http://www.correctionsone.com/corrections/articles/7527475-15-prison-tattoos-and-their-meanings/

Covington, S.S., & Bloom, B.E. (2006). Gender responsive treatment and services in correctional settings. *Women and Therapy, 29* (3), 9-33.

Craissati, J., Minoidis, P., Shaw, J., Chuan, A. J., Simons, S., Joseph, N. (2011). *Working with personality disordered offenders: A practitioner's guide.* Ministry of Justice National Offender Management Program. Retrieved from https://www.justice.gov.uk/downloads/offenders/mentally-disordered-offenders/working-with-personality-disordered-offenders.pdf

Department of Justice. (2011). *Police use of force, tasers and other less-lethal weapons.* Retrieved from https://www.ncjrs.gov/pdffiles1/nij/232215.pdf

Deitch, M. (2009) *From time out to hard time: Young children in the adult criminal justice system.* Austin, TX: The University of Texas at Austin, LBJ School of Public Affairs Retrieved from

References

http://www.utexas.edu/lbj/archive/news/images/file/From%20Time%20Out%20to%20Hard%20Time-revised%20final.pdf

Fry, S. T., & Johnstone, M. J. (2008). *Ethics in nursing practice: A guide to ethical decision making* (3rd ed.) Oxford, UK: International Council of Nurses-Blackwell Publishing.

Glaze, L. E., & James, D. J. (2006). Mental health problems of prison and jail inmates. *Bureau of Justice Statistics Special Report.* Retrieved from http://www.bjs.gov/content/pub/pdf/mhppji.pdf

Greenberg, E., Dunleavy, E., & Kutner, M. (2007). *Literacy behind bars: Results from the 2003 National Assessment of Adult Literacy Prison Survey.* U.S. Department of Education. Retrieved from http://nces.ed.gov/pubs2007/2007473.pdf

Guido, G. W. (2011). Legal and ethical issues. In P. S. Yoder-Wise (Ed.), *Leading and managing in nursing* (5th ed.), St. Louis, MO: Elsevier Mosby.

Guthrie, B. J. (2011). Toward a gender-responsive restorative correctional health care model. *Journal of Obstetric, Gynecologic and Neonatal Nurses, 40*, 497-505.

Hardesty, K. N., Champion, D. R., & Champion, J. E. (2007). Nail nurses: Perceptions, stigmatization, and working styles in correctional health care. *Journal of Correctional Health Care, 13*, 196-205.

Harmon, R. E. (2013). Mental health. In L. Schoenly & C. M. Knox (Eds.), *Essentials of correctional nursing* (pp. 221-245). New York, NY: Springer.

Hayes, L. (2010). *National study of jail suicide: 20 years later.* Retrieved from http://static.nicic.gov/Library/024308.pdf

Hoffman, P. (2009). Health care legal concepts. In R. Carroll (Ed.), *Risk management handbook for health care organizations* (Student ed., pp. 115-157). San Francisco, CA: Jossey-Bass.

International Council of Nurses (ICN). (2011). *Position statement: Nurses' role in the care of detainees and prisoners.* Retrieved from http://www.icn.ch/images/stories/documents/publications/position_statements/A13_Nurses_Role_Detainees_Prisoners.pdf

Knox, C. (2013). Dental conditions. In L. Schoenly & C. M. Knox (Eds.), *Essentials of correctional nursing* (pp. 123-40). New York, NY: Springer.

Lachman, V. D. (2007). Moral courage: A virtue in need of development? *MedSurg Nursing, 16*(2), 31-33. Retrieved from http://www.nursingworld.org/MainMenuCategories/EthicsStandards/Courage-and-Distress/Moral-Courage-A-Virtue-in-Need-of-Development.pdf

Lachman, V. D. (2008). Whistleblowers: Troublemakers or virtuous nurses? *MedSurg Nursing, 17*(2), 126-134. Retrieved from http://www.nursingworld.org/documentvault/ethics/whistleblowers-.pdf

Lachman, V. D. (2010). Strategies necessary for moral courage. *OJIN: The Online Journal of Issues in Nursing, 15*(3). Man. 3. doi: 10.3912/OJIN.Vol15No03Man03

Maroney, M. K. (2005). Caring and custody: Two faces of the same reality. *Journal of Correctional Health Care, 11*(1), 157-169.

McCarthy, D. H. (2013). Learning common categories of malpractice claims against nurses and how to reduce potential liability. *ADVANCE Healthcare Network*. Retrieved from http://nursing.advanceweb.com/Continuing-Education/CE-Articles/Is-It-Malpractice.aspx

Moore, J. (2013). Legal considerations in correctional nursing. In L. Schoenly & C. M. Knox (Eds.), *Essentials of correctional nursing* (pp. 327-348). New York, NY: Springer.

National Commission on Correctional Health Care (U.S.). (2014). *Standards for health services in prisons, 2014.* Chicago, IL: National Commission on Correctional Health Care.

National Commission on Correctional Health Care (NCCHC). (July, 2014). *Nurses' scope of practice and delegation authority.* Retrieved from http://www.ncchc.org/filebin/Resources/Nurses-Scope-2014.pdf

National Commission on Correctional Health Care (NCCHC). (2014). *Women's health care in correctional settings. NCCHC Position Statements.* Retrieved from http://www.ncchc.org/women%E2%80%99s-health-care

National Council of State Boards of Nursing (NCSBN). (2014). *The nurse's guide to professional boundaries.* Retrieved from https://www.ncsbn.org/ProfessionalBoundaries_Complete.pdf

Nursing Service Organization. (2011). *Understanding nursing liability, 2006-2010. A 3-part approach.* Retrieved from http://www.nso.com/pdfs/db/RN-2010-CNA-Claims-Study.pdf?fileName=RN-2010-CNA-Claims-Study.pdf&folder=pdfs/db&isLiveStr=Y

References

Puisis, M. (2006). *Clinical practice in correctional medicine*. Philadelphia, PA: Mosby Elsevier.

Reeves, R. R., Parker, J. D., & Burke, R. S. (2010). Unrecognized physical illness prompting psychiatric admission. *Annals of Clinical Psychiatry, 22*(3), 180-185.

Samuel, E., Williams, R. B., & Ferrell, R, B. (2009). Excited delirium: Consideration of selected medical and psychiatric issues. *Neuropsychiatric Disease and Treatment, 5*, 61–66.

Schoenly, L. (2013). Context of correctional nursing. In L. Schoenly & C. M. Knox (Eds.), *Essentials of correctional nursing* (pp. 1–18). New York, NY: Springer.

Schoenly, L. (2013). Ethical principles of correctional nursing. In L. Schoenly & C. M. Knox (Eds.), *Essentials of correctional nursing* (pp. 19-37). New York, NY: Springer.

Schoenly, L. (2013). Safety for the nurse and the patient. In L. Schoenly & C. M. Knox (Eds.), *Essentials of correctional nursing* (pp. 55-79). New York, NY: Springer.

Schoenly, L. (2014). *Correctional health care patient safety handbook: Reduce clinical error, manage risk, and improve quality*. Nashville, TN: Enchanted Mountain Press.

Shiroma, J. J., Ferguson, P. L., & Pickelsimer, E. E. (2010). Prevalence of traumatic brain injury in an offender population: A meta-analysis. *Journal of Correctional Health Care, 16*(2), 147-159.

Smith, C. G., & Stopford, W. (1999). Health hazards of pepper spray. *North Carolina Medical Journal, 60*(5), 268-274. Retrieved from http://duketox.mc.duke.edu/pepper%20spray.pdf

Sportsman, S., & Hamilton, P. (2007). Conflict management styles in nursing and allied health professionals. *Journal of Professional Nursing, 23*(3), 157-166.

Tapia, N. D., & Vaughn, M. S. (2010). Legal issues regarding medical care for pregnant inmates. *The Prison Journal, 90*(4), 417-446.

The National Center on Addiction and Substance Abuse at Columbia University. (2010). *Behind bars II: Substance abuse and America's prison population*. New York, NY: The National Center on Addiction and Substance Abuse at Columbia University. Retrieved from http://www.casacolumbia.org/addiction-research/reports/substance-abuse-prison-system-2010

Torrey, E. F., Kennard, A. D., Eslinger, D., Lamb, R., & Pavle, J. (2010). *More mentally ill persons are in jails and prisons than hospitals: A survey of the states.* Treatment Advocacy Center: National Sheriffs' Association. Retrieved from http://tacreports.org/storage/documents/2010-jail-study.pdf

Treasurer, B. (2008). *Courage goes to work: How to build backbones, boost performance, and get results.* San Francisco, CA: Berrett-Koehler Publishers.

Wakefield, D. S. & Wakefield, B. J. (2009). Are verbal orders a threat to patient safety? *Quality Safety Health Care, 18*(3), 165-8. doi:10.1136/qshc.2009.034041

Watson, J. (2012). *Human caring science: A theory of nursing* (2nd ed.). Boston, MA: Jones & Bartlett.

Weiskopf, C. S. (2005). *Nurses' experience of caring for inmate patients. Journal of Advanced Nursing, 49*(4), 336-343.

Wilper, A. P., Woolhandler, S., Boyd, J. W., Lasswer, K. E., McCormick, D., Bor, D. H., & Himmelstein, D. U. (2009). The health and health care of US prisoners: Results of a nationwide survey. *American Journal of Public Health, 99*(4), 666-672.